The Vibrant Pegan Diet Cookbook for Beginners

Boost your Health and Live better with these Super Easy and Affordable Pegan Recipes

Emy Fit

© Copyright 2020 - All rights reserved.

The content contained within this book may not be reproduced, duplicated or transmitted without direct written permission from the author or the publisher.

Under no circumstances will any blame or legal responsibility be held against the publisher, or author, for any damages, reparation, or monetary loss due to the information contained within this book. Either directly or indirectly.

Legal Notice:

This book is copyright protected. This book is only for personal use. You cannot amend, distribute, sell, use, quote or paraphrase any part, or the content within this book, without the consent of the author or publisher.

Disclaimer Notice:

Please note the information contained within this document is for educational and entertainment purposes only. All effort has been executed to present accurate, up to date, and reliable, complete information. No warranties of any kind are declared or implied. Readers acknowledge that the author is not engaging in the rendering of legal, financial, medical or professional advice. The content within this book has been derived from various sources. Please consult a licensed professional before attempting any techniques outlined in this book.

By reading this document, the reader agrees that under no circumstances is the author responsible for any losses, direct or indirect, which are incurred as a result of the use of information contained within this document, including, but not limited to, — errors, omissions, or inaccuracies.

Table of Contents

Mediterranean Eggs 11

Pastry-Less Spanakopita 13

Date and Walnut Overnight Oats 14

Greek Quinoa Breakfast Bowl 15

Mediterranean Frittata... 17

Honey-Caramelized Figs with Greek Yogurt 19

Savory Quinoa Egg Muffins with Spinach 21

Avocado Tomato Gouda Socca Pizza.. 23

Sunny-Side Up Baked Eggs with Swiss Chard, Feta, and Basil 25

Polenta with Sautéed Chard and Fried Eggs 27

Smoked Salmon Egg Scramble with Dill and Chives....................................... 29

Classic Lentil Soup with Swiss Chard 31

Spicy Winter Farro Soup.. 33

Rainbow Chickpea Salad 35

Mediterranean-Style Lentil Salad 36

Roasted Asparagus and Avocado Salad... 38

Creamed Green Bean Salad with Pine Nuts.. 40

Cannellini Bean Soup with Kale 41

Hearty Cream of Mushroom Soup 43

Authentic Italian Panzanella Salad 46

Quinoa and Black Bean Salad... 49

Rich Bulgur Salad with Herbs 51

Classic Roasted Pepper Salad 53

Hearty Winter Quinoa Soup... 54

Green Lentil Salad 56

Acorn Squash, Chickpea and Couscous Soup... 58

Cabbage Soup with Garlic Crostini 62

Cream of Green Bean Soup 65

Traditional French Onion Soup.. 68

Roasted Carrot Soup 69

Italian Penne Pasta Salad 72

Arugula with Fruits and Nuts 73

Broccoli Salad 74

Brunoise Salad 75

Breakfast Sandwich 80

Turkey Breakfast Sandwich 81

Eggplant Breakfast Spread 83

Chicken Liver Breakfast Spread 85

Mushroom Spread 86

Breakfast Chia Pudding 88

Breakfast Sweet Potatoes 89

Eggs with Zucchini Noodles 90

Smoked Salmon and Poached Eggs on Toast 92

Mediterranean Breakfast Salad 94

Honey Almond Ricotta Spread with Peaches 96

Mediterranean Eggs Cups 98

Low-Carb Baked Eggs with Avocado and Feta 100

Mediterranean Eggs White Breakfast Sandwich with Roasted Tomatoes .. 102

Greek Yogurt Pancakes 103

Mediterranean Feta and Quinoa Egg Muffins 105

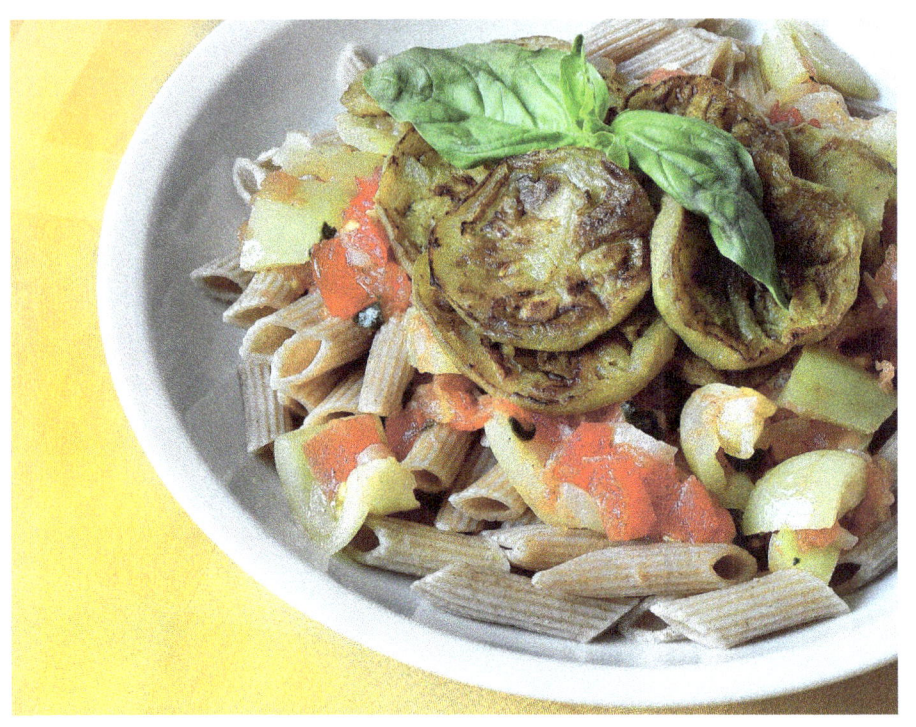

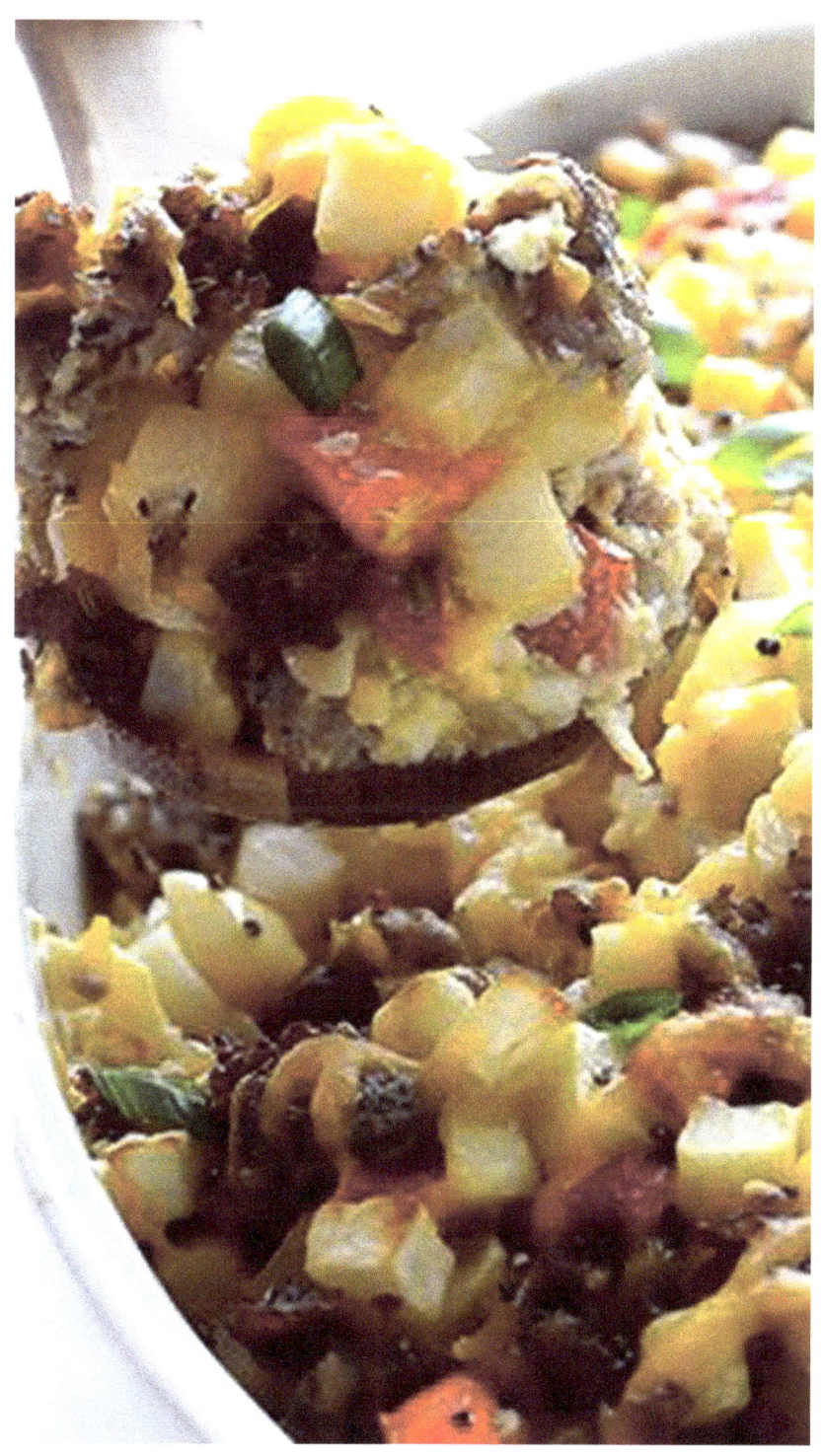

Mediterranean Eggs

Preparation Time: 15 Minutes
Cooking Time: 20 Minutes
Servings: 2
Ingredients:

- 5 tbsp. of divided olive oil
- 2 diced medium-sized Spanish onions
- 2 diced red bell peppers
- 2 minced cloves garlic
- 1 teaspoon cumin seeds
- 4 diced large ripe tomatoes
- 1 tablespoon of honey
- Salt
- Freshly ground black pepper
- 1/3 cup crumbled feta
- 4 eggs
- 1 teaspoon zaatar spice
  Grilled pita during serving

Directions:

1. To start with, you have to add 3 tablespoons of olive oil into a pan and heat it over medium heat. Along with the oil, sauté the cumin seeds, onions, garlic, and red pepper for a few minutes.
2. After that, add the diced tomatoes and salt and pepper to taste and cook them for about 10 minutes till they come together and form a light sauce.
3. With that, half the preparation is already done. Now you just have to break the eggs directly into the sauce and poach them. However, you must keep in mind to cook the egg whites but keep the yolks still runny. This takes about 8 to 10 minutes.
4. While plating adds some feta and olive oil with zaatar spice to further enhance the flavors. Once done, serve with grilled pita.

Nutrition:
Calories: 304
Protein: 12 g
Fat: 16 g
Carbs: 28 g

Pastry-Less Spanakopita

Preparation Time: 5 Minutes
Cooking Time: 20 Minutes
Servings: 4
Ingredients:

- 1/8 teaspoons black pepper, add as per taste
- 1/3 cup of virgin olive oil
- 4 lightly beaten eggs
- 7 cups of Lettuce, preferably a spring mix (mesclun)
- 1/2 cup of crumbled Feta cheese
- 1/8 teaspoon of Sea salt, add to taste
- 1 finely chopped medium Yellow onion

Directions:

1. For this delicious recipe, you need to first start by preheating the oven to 180C and grease the flan dish.
2. Once done, pour the extra virgin olive oil into a large saucepan and heat it over medium heat with the onions, until they are translucent. To that, add greens and keep stirring until all the ingredients are wilted.
3. After completing that, you should season it with salt and pepper and transfer the greens to the prepared dish and sprinkle on some feta cheese.
4. Pour the eggs and bake it for 20 minutes till it is cooked through and slightly brown.

Nutrition:

Calories: 325

Protein: 11.2 g

Fat: 27.9 g

Carbs: 7.3 g

Date and Walnut Overnight Oats

Preparation Time: 5 Minutes

Cooking Time: 20 Minutes

Servings: 2

Ingredients:

- ¼ Cup Greek Yogurt, Plain
- 1/3 cup of yogurt
- 2/3 cup of oats
- 1 cup of milk
- 2 tsp date syrup or you can also use maple syrup or honey
- 1 mashed banana
- ¼ tsp cinnamon
- ¼ cup walnuts
- pinch of salt (approx.1/8 tsp)

Directions:

1. Firstly, get a mason jar or a small bowl and add all the ingredients.
2. After that stir and mix all the ingredients well.
3. Cover it securely, and cool it in a refrigerator overnight.
4. After that, take it out the next morning, add more liquid or cinnamon if required, and serve cold. (However, you can also microwave it for people with a warmer palate.)

Nutrition:

Calories: 350

Protein: 14 g

Fat: 12 g

Carbs: 49 g

Greek Quinoa Breakfast Bowl

Preparation Time: 10 Minutes
Cooking Time: 20 Minutes
Servings: 2
Ingredients:

- 2 large eggs
- 3/4 cup Greek yogurt
- 2 cups of cooked quinoa
- 3/4 cup muhammara
- 3 ounces of baby spinach
- 4 ounces of marinated kalamata olives
- 6 ounces of sliced cherry tomatoes
- 1 halved lemon
- hot chili oil
- salt & pepper to taste
- fresh dill and sesame seeds to garnish

Directions:

1. Add all the ingredients, Greek yogurt, granulated garlic, onion powder, salt, and pepper, and whisk them all together and set aside.
2. In a different large saucepan, heat the olive oil on medium-high heat and add the spinach. You have to keep in mind to cook the spinach till it is slightly wilted. This takes about 3-4 minutes.
3. After that, cook the cherry tomatoes in the same skillet for 3-4 minutes till they are softened.
4. Stir in the egg mixture into this for about 7 to 9 minutes, until it has set and cooked them so that they get scrambled.
5. After the eggs have set, stir in the quinoa and feta and cook until it is heated all the way through and serve it hot with some fresh dill and sesame seeds to garnish.

Nutrition:
Calories: 357
Protein: 23 g
Fat: 20 g
Carbs: 20 g

Mediterranean Frittata

Preparation Time: 8 Minutes
Cooking Time: 6 Minutes
Servings: 4
Ingredients:

- Two teaspoons of olive oil
- 3/4 cup of baby spinach, packed
- Two green onions
- Four egg whites, large
- Six large eggs
  1/3 cup of crumbled feta cheese, (1.3 ounces) along with sun-dried tomatoes
- and basil Two teaspoons of salt-free
- Greek seasoning 1/4 teaspoon of salt
-

Directions:

1. Take a boiler and preheat it
2. Take a ten-inch ovenproof skillet and pour the oil into it and keep the skillet on a medium flame.
3. While the oil gets heated, chop the spinach roughly and the onions.
4. Put the eggs, egg whites, Greek seasoning, cheese, as well as salt in a large mixing bowl and mix it thoroughly using a whisker.
5. Add the chopped spinach and onions into the mixing bowl and stir it well.
6. Pour the mixture into the pan and cook it for 2 minutes or more until the edges of the mixture set well. Lift the edges of the mixture gently and tilt the pan so that the uncooked portion can get underneath it. Cook for additional two minutes so that the whole mixture gets cooked properly.
7. Broil for two to three minutes till the center gets set.
8. Your Frittata is now ready. Serve it hot by cutting it into four wedges.

Nutrition:

Calories: 178

Protein: 16 g

Fat: 12 g

Carbs: 2.2 g

Honey-Caramelized Figs with Greek Yogurt

Preparation Time: 5 Minutes
Cooking Time: 5 Minutes
Servings: 4
Ingredients:

- Four fresh halved figs
- Two tablespoons of melted butter, 30ml
- Two tablespoons of brown sugar, 30ml
- Two cups of Greek yogurt 500ml
 1/4 cup of honey, 60ml

Directions:

1. Take a non-stick skillet and preheat it over a medium flame
2. Put the butter on the pan and toss the figs into it and sprinkle in some brown sugar over it.
3. Put the figs on the pan and cut off the side of the figs.
4. Cook the figs on a medium flame for 2-3 minutes until they turn a golden brown.
5. Turn over the figs and cook them for 2-3 minutes again
6. Remove the figs from the pan and let it cool down a little.
7. Take a plate and put a scoop of Greek yogurt on it. Put the cooked figs over the yogurts and drizzle the honey over it

Nutrition:

Calories: 350

Protein: 6 g

Fat: 19 g

Carbs: 40 g

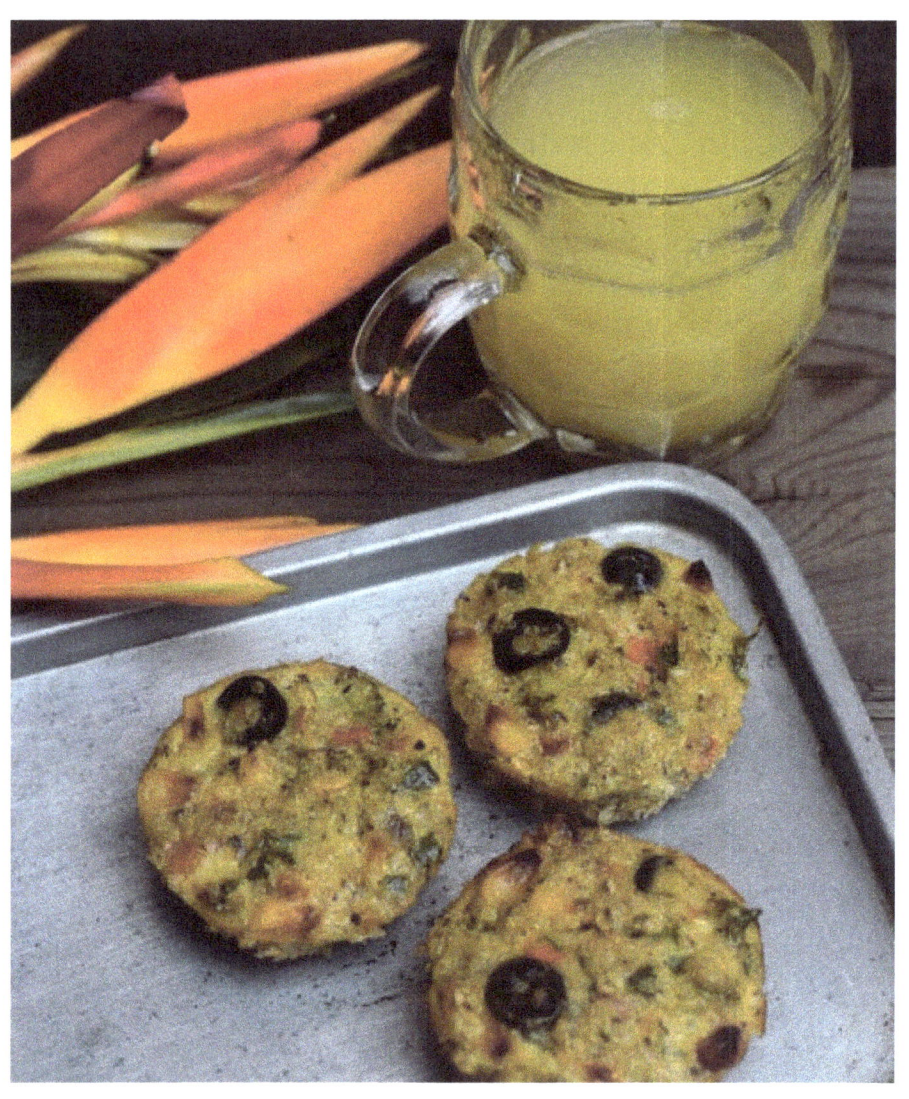

Savory Quinoa Egg Muffins with Spinach

Preparation Time: 15 Minutes

Cooking Time: 20 Minutes

Servings: 2

Ingredients:

- One cup of quinoa
- Two cups of water/ vegetable broth)
- Four ounces of spinach which is about one cup
- Half chopped onion
- Two whole eggs
- 1/4 cup of grated cheese
- Half teaspoon of oregano or thyme
- Half teaspoon of garlic powder
- Half teaspoon of salt

Directions:

1. Take a medium saucepan and put water in it. Add the quinoa in the water and bring the whole thing to a simmer. Cover the pan and cook it for 10 minutes till the water gets absorbed by the quinoa. Remove the saucepan from the heat and let it cool down.
2. Take a nonstick pan and heat the onions till they turn soft and then add spinach. Cook all of them together till the spinach gets a little wilted and then remove it from the heat.
3. Preheat the oven to 176.667 C
4. Take a muffin pan and grease it lightly
5. Take a large bowl and add the cooked quinoa along with the cooked onions, spinach, and add cheese, eggs, thyme or oregano, salt, garlic powder, pepper and mix them together.
6. Put a spoonful of the mixture into a muffin tin. Make sure it is ¼ of a cup.

7. In the preheated pan, put it in the pan and bake it for around 20 minutes.

Nutrition:

Calories: 61

Protein: 4 g

Fat: 3 g

Carbs: 6 g

Avocado Tomato Gouda Socca Pizza

Preparation Time: 20 Minutes

Cooking Time: 20 Minutes

Servings: 2

Ingredients:

- One and 1/4 cups of chickpea or garbanzo bean flour
- One and 1/4 cups of cold water
- 1/4 teaspoon of pepper and sea salt each
- Two teaspoons of avocado or olive oil. Take one teaspoon extra for heating the pan
- One teaspoon of minced Garlic which will be around two cloves
- One teaspoon of Onion powder/other herb seasoning powder
- Ten to twelve-inch cast iron pan
- One sliced tomato
- Half avocado
- Two ounces of thinly sliced Gouda
- 1/4-1/3 cup of Tomato sauce
- Two or three teaspoons of chopped green scallion/onion
- Sprouted greens for green
- Extra pepper/salt for sprinkling on top of the pizza
- Red pepper flakes

Directions:

1. Mix the flour with two teaspoons of olive oil, herbs, water, and whisk it until a smooth mixture form. Keep it at room temperature for around 15-20 minutes to let the batter settle
2. In the meantime, preheat the oven and place the pan inside the oven and let it get heated for around 10 minutes
3. When the pan gets preheated, chop up the vegetables into fine slices
4. Remove the pan after ten minutes using oven mitts

5. Put one teaspoon of oil and swirl it all around to coat the pan
6. Pour the batter into the pan then slant the pan so that the batter spreads evenly throughout the pan.
7. Turn down the over to 425f and place back the pan for 5-8 minutes
8. Remove the pan from the oven and add the sliced avocado, tomato and on top of that, add the gouda slices and the onion slices
9. Put the pizza into the oven then wait till the cheese get melted or the sides of the bread gets crusty and brown
10. Remove the pizza from the pan and add the microgreens on top, along with the toppings.

Nutrition:

Calories: 416

Protein: 15 g

Fat: 10 g

Carbs: 37 g

Sunny-Side Up Baked Eggs with Swiss Chard, Feta, and Basil

Preparation Time: 15 Minutes

Cooking Time: 10 Minutes

Servings: 4

Ingredients:

- 4 bell peppers, any color
- 1 tablespoon extra-virgin olive oil
- 8 large eggs
  ¾ teaspoon kosher salt, divided
- ¼ teaspoon freshly ground black pepper, divided
- 1 avocado, peeled, pitted, and diced
- ¼ cup red onion, diced
- ¼ cup fresh basil, chopped
- Juice of ½ lime

Directions:

1. Stem and seed the bell peppers. Cut 2 (2-inch-thick) rings from each pepper. Chop the remaining bell pepper into small dice and set aside.
2. Heat the olive oil in a large skillet over medium heat. Add 4 bell pepper rings, then crack 1 egg in the middle of each ring. Season with ¼ teaspoon of the salt and 1/8 teaspoon of the black pepper. Cook until the egg whites are generally set, but the yolks are still runny 2 to 3 minutes. Gently flip and cook 1 additional minute for over easy. Move the egg–bell pepper rings to a platter or onto plates and repeats with the remaining 4 bell pepper rings.
3. In a medium bowl, blend the avocado, onion, basil, lime juice, reserved diced bell pepper, the remaining ¼ teaspoon kosher salt, and the remaining 1/8 teaspoon black pepper. Divide among the 4 plates.

Nutrition:

Calories: 270

Protein: 15 g
Fat: 19 g
Carbs: 12 g

Polenta with Sautéed Chard and Fried Eggs

Preparation Time: 5 Minutes

Cooking Time: 20 Minutes

Servings: 4

Ingredients:

- 2½ cups water
- ½ teaspoon kosher salt
- ¾ cups whole-grain cornmeal
- ¼ teaspoon freshly ground black pepper
- 2 tablespoons grated Parmesan cheese
- 1 tablespoon extra-virgin olive oil
- 1 bunch (about 6 ounces) Swiss chard, leaves and stems chopped and separated
- 2 garlic cloves, sliced
- ¼ teaspoon kosher salt
- 1/8 teaspoon freshly ground black pepper
- Lemon juice (optional)
- 1 tablespoon extra-virgin olive oil
- 4 large eggs

Directions:

TO MAKE THE POLENTA

1. Le the water and salt to boil in a medium saucepan over high heat. Slowly add the cornmeal, whisking constantly.
2. Decrease the heat to low, cover, and cook for 10 to 15 minutes, stirring often to avoid lumps. Stir in the pepper and Parmesan and divide among 4 bowls.

TO MAKE THE CHARD

1. Heat the oil in a large frying pan on medium heat. Add the chard stems, garlic, salt, and pepper; sauté for 2 minutes. Add the chard leaves and cook until wilted, about 3 to 5 minutes.

2. Add a spritz of lemon juice (if desired), toss together, and divide evenly on top of the polenta.

TO MAKE THE EGGS

1. Heat the oil in the same large skillet over medium-high heat. Crack each egg into the skillet, taking care not to crowd the skillet and leaving space between the eggs. Cook until the whites are set and golden around the edges, about 2 to 3 minutes.
2. Serve sunny-side up or flip the eggs over carefully and cook 1 minute longer for over easy. Put one egg on top of the polenta and chard in each bowl.

Nutrition:

Calories: 310

Protein: 17 g

Fat: 18 g

Carbs: 21 g

Smoked Salmon Egg Scramble with Dill and Chives

Preparation Time: 5 Minutes

Cooking Time: 5 Minutes

Servings: 2

Ingredients:

- 4 large eggs
- 1 tablespoon milk
- 1 tablespoon fresh chives, minced
- 1 tablespoon fresh dill, minced
- ¼ teaspoon kosher salt
- 1/8 teaspoon freshly ground black pepper
- 2 teaspoons extra-virgin olive oil
- 2 ounces smoked salmon, thinly sliced

Directions:

1. In a large bowl, blend together the eggs, milk, chives, dill, salt, and pepper.
2. Heat the olive oil in a medium skillet or sauté pan over medium heat. Add the egg mixture and cook for about 3 minutes, stirring occasionally.
3. Add the salmon and cook until the eggs are set but moist about 1 minute.

Nutrition:

Calories: 325

Protein: 23 g

Fat: 26 g

Carbs: 1 g

Soup and Salad Recipes

Classic Lentil Soup with Swiss Chard

Preparation time: 10 minutes
Cooking Time: 25 minutes
Servings: 5
Ingredients:

- 2 tablespoons olive oil
- 1 white onion, chopped
- 1 teaspoon garlic, minced
- 2 large carrots, chopped
- 1 parsnip, chopped
- 2 stalks celery, chopped
- 2 bay leaves
- 1/2 teaspoon dried thyme
- 1/4 teaspoon ground cumin
- 5 cups roasted vegetable broth
- 1 ¼ cups brown lentils, soaked overnight and rinsed
- 2 cups Swiss chard, torn into pieces

Directions:

1. In a heavy-bottomed pot, heat the olive oil over a moderate heat. Now, sauté the vegetables along with the spices for about 3 minutes until they are just tender.
2. Add in the vegetable broth and lentils, bringing it to a boil. Immediately turn the heat to a simmer and add in the bay leaves. Let it cook for about 15 minutes or until lentils are tender.
3. Add in the Swiss chard, cover and let it simmer for 5 minutes more or until the chard wilts.
4. Serve in individual bowls and enjoy!

Nutrition: Calories: 148; Fat: 7.2g; Carbs: 14.6g; Protein: 7.7g

Spicy Winter Farro Soup

Preparation time: 10 minutes
Cooking Time: 30 minutes
Servings: 4
Ingredients:

- 2 tablespoons olive oil
- 1 medium-sized leek, chopped
- 1 medium-sized turnip, sliced
- 2 Italian peppers, seeded and chopped
- 1 jalapeno pepper, minced
- 2 potatoes, peeled and diced
- 4 cups vegetable broth
- 1 cup farro, rinsed
- 1/2 teaspoon granulated garlic
- 1/2 teaspoon turmeric powder
- 1 bay laurel
- 2 cups spinach, turn into pieces

Directions:

1. In a heavy-bottomed pot, heat the olive oil over a moderate heat. Now, sauté the leek, turnip, peppers and potatoes for about 5 minutes until they are crisp-tender.
2. Add in the vegetable broth, farro, granulated garlic, turmeric and bay laurel; bring it to a boil.
3. Immediately turn the heat to a simmer. Let it cook for about 25 minutes or until farro and potatoes have softened.
4. Add in the spinach and remove the pot from the heat; let the spinach sit in the residual heat until it wilts. Bon appétit!

Nutrition: Calories: 298; Fat: 8.9g; Carbs: 44.6g; Protein: 11.7g

Rainbow Chickpea Salad

Preparation time: 10 minutes
Cooking Time: 30 minutes
Servings: 4
Ingredients:

- 16 ounces canned chickpeas, drained
- 1 medium avocado, sliced
- 1 bell pepper, seeded and sliced
- 1 large tomato, sliced
- 2 cucumber, diced
- 1 red onion, sliced
- 1/2 teaspoon garlic, minced
- 1/4 cup fresh parsley, chopped
- 1/4 cup olive oil
- 2 tablespoons apple cider vinegar
- 1/2 lime, freshly squeezed
- Sea salt and ground black pepper, to taste

Directions:

1. Toss all the Ingredients in a salad bowl.
2. Place the salad in your refrigerator for about 1 hour before serving.
3. Bon appétit!

Nutrition: Calories: 378; Fat: 24g; Carbs: 34.2g; Protein: 10.1g

Mediterranean-Style Lentil Salad

Preparation time: 10 minutes
Cooking Time: 20 minutes + chilling time
Servings: 5
Ingredients:

- 1 ½ cups red lentil, rinsed
- 1 teaspoon deli mustard
- 1/2 lemon, freshly squeezed
- 2 tablespoons tamari sauce
- 2 scallion stalks, chopped
- 1/4 cup extra-virgin olive oil
- 2 garlic cloves, minced
- 1 cup butterhead lettuce, torn into pieces
- 2 tablespoons fresh parsley, chopped
- 2 tablespoons fresh cilantro, chopped
- 1 teaspoon fresh basil
- 1 teaspoon fresh oregano
- 1 ½ cups cherry tomatoes, halved
- 3 ounces Kalamata olives, pitted and halved

Directions:

1. In a large-sized saucepan, bring 4 ½ cups of the water and the red lentils to a boil.
2. Immediately turn the heat to a simmer and continue to cook your lentils for about 15 minutes or until tender. Drain and let it cool completely.
3. Transfer the lentils to a salad bowl; toss the lentils with the remaining Ingredients until well combined.
4. Serve chilled or at room temperature. Bon appétit!

Nutrition: Calories: 348; Fat: 15g; Carbs: 41.6g; Protein: 15.8g

Roasted Asparagus and Avocado Salad

Preparation time: 10 minutes
Cooking Time: 20 minutes + chilling time
Servings: 4
Ingredients:

- 1 pound asparagus, trimmed, cut into bite-sized pieces
- 1 white onion, chopped
- 2 garlic cloves, minced
- 1 Roma tomato, sliced
- 1/4 cup olive oil
- 1/4 cup balsamic vinegar
- 1 tablespoon stone-ground mustard
- 2 tablespoons fresh parsley, chopped
- 1 tablespoon fresh cilantro, chopped
- 1 tablespoon fresh basil, chopped
- Sea salt and ground black pepper, to taste
- 1 small avocado, pitted and diced
- 1/2 cup pine nuts, roughly chopped

Directions:
1. Begin by preheating your oven to 420 degrees F.
2. Toss the asparagus with 1 tablespoon of the olive oil and arrange them on a parchment-lined roasting pan.
3. Bake for about 15 minutes, rotating the pan once or twice to promote even cooking. Let it cool completely and place in your salad bowl.
4. Toss the asparagus with the vegetables, olive oil, vinegar, mustard and herbs. Salt and pepper to taste.
5. Toss to combine and top with avocado and pine nuts. Bon appétit!

Nutrition: Calories: 378; Fat: 33.2g; Carbs: 18.6g; Protein: 7.8g

Creamed Green Bean Salad with Pine Nuts

Preparation time: 10 minutes
Cooking Time: 10 minutes + chilling time
Servings: 5
Ingredients:

- 1 ½ pounds green beans, trimmed
- 2 medium tomatoes, diced
- 2 bell peppers, seeded and diced
- 4 tablespoons shallots, chopped
- 1/2 cup pine nuts, roughly chopped
- 1/2 cup vegan mayonnaise
- 1 tablespoon deli mustard
- 2 tablespoons fresh basil, chopped
- 2 tablespoons fresh parsley, chopped
- 1/2 teaspoon red pepper flakes, crushed
- Sea salt and freshly ground black pepper, to taste

Directions:

1. Boil the green beans in a large saucepan of salted water until they are just tender or about 2 minutes.
2. Drain and let the beans cool completely; then, transfer them to a salad bowl. Toss the beans with the remaining ingredients.
3. Taste and adjust the seasonings. Bon appétit!

Nutrition: Calories: 308; Fat: 26.2g; Carbs: 16.6g; Protein: 5.8g

Cannellini Bean Soup with Kale

Preparation time: 10 minutes
Cooking Time: 25 minutes
Servings: 5
Ingredients:

- 1 tablespoon olive oil
- 1/2 teaspoon ginger, minced
- 1/2 teaspoon cumin seeds
- 1 red onion, chopped
- 1 carrot, trimmed and chopped
- 1 parsnip, trimmed and chopped
- 2 garlic cloves, minced
- 5 cups vegetable broth
- 12 ounces Cannellini beans, drained
- 2 cups kale, torn into pieces
- Sea salt and ground black pepper, to taste

Directions:

1. In a heavy-bottomed pot, heat the olive over medium-high heat. Now, sauté the ginger and cumin for 1 minute or so.
2. Now, add in the onion, carrot and parsnip; continue sautéing an additional 3 minutes or until the vegetables are just tender.
3. Add in the garlic and continue to sauté for 1 minute or until aromatic.
4. Then, pour in the vegetable broth and bring to a boil. Immediately reduce the heat to a simmer and let it cook for 10 minutes.
5. Fold in the Cannellini beans and kale; continue to simmer until the kale wilts and everything is

thoroughly heated. Season with salt and pepper to taste.
6. Ladle into individual bowls and serve hot. Bon appétit!

Nutrition: Calories: 188; Fat: 4.7g; Carbs: 24.5g; Protein: 11.1g

Hearty Cream of Mushroom Soup

Preparation time: 10 minutes
Cooking Time: 15 minutes
Servings: 5
Ingredients:

- 2 tablespoons soy butter
- 1 large shallot, chopped
- 20 ounces Cremini mushrooms, sliced
- 2 cloves garlic, minced
- 4 tablespoons flaxseed meal
- 5 cups vegetable broth
- 1 1/3 cups full-fat coconut milk
- 1 bay leaf
- Sea salt and ground black pepper, to taste

Directions:

1. In a stockpot, melt the vegan butter over medium-high heat. Once hot, cook the shallot for about 3 minutes until tender and fragrant.
2. Add in the mushrooms and garlic and continue cooking until the mushrooms have softened. Add in the flaxseed meal and continue to cook for 1 minute or so.
3. Add in the remaining ingredients. Let it simmer, covered and continue to cook for 5 to 6 minutes more until your soup has thickened slightly.
4. Bon appétit!

Nutrition: Calories: 308; Fat: 25.5g; Carbs: 11.8g; Protein: 11.6g

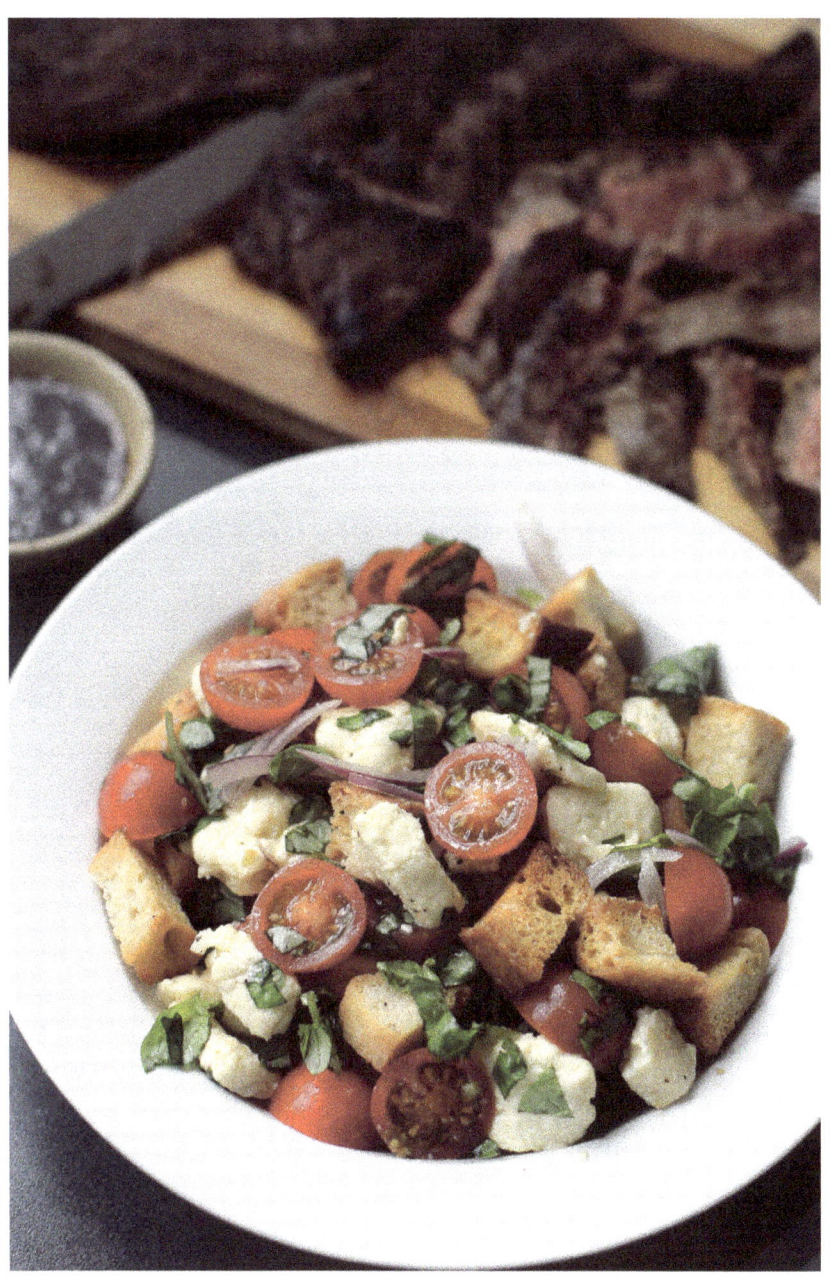

Authentic Italian Panzanella Salad

Preparation time: 10 minutes
Cooking Time: 35 minutes
Servings: 3
Ingredients:

- 3 cups artisan bread, broken into 1-inch cubes
- 3/4-pound asparagus, trimmed and cut into bite-sized pieces
- 4 tablespoons extra-virgin olive oil
- 1 red onion, chopped
- 2 tablespoons fresh lime juice
- 1 teaspoon deli mustard
- 2 medium heirloom tomatoes, diced
- 2 cups arugula
- 2 cups baby spinach
- 2 Italian peppers, seeded and sliced
- Sea salt and ground black pepper, to taste

Directions:

1. Arrange the bread cubes on a parchment-lined baking sheet. Bake in the preheated oven at 310 degrees F for about 20 minutes, rotating the baking sheet twice during the baking time; reserve.
2. Turn the oven to 420 degrees F and toss the asparagus with 1 tablespoon of olive oil. Roast the asparagus for about 15 minutes or until crisp-tender.

3. Toss the remaining Ingredients in a salad bowl; top with the roasted asparagus and toasted bread.
4. Bon appétit!

Nutrition: Calories: 334; Fat: 20.4g; Carbs: 33.3g; Protein: 8.3g

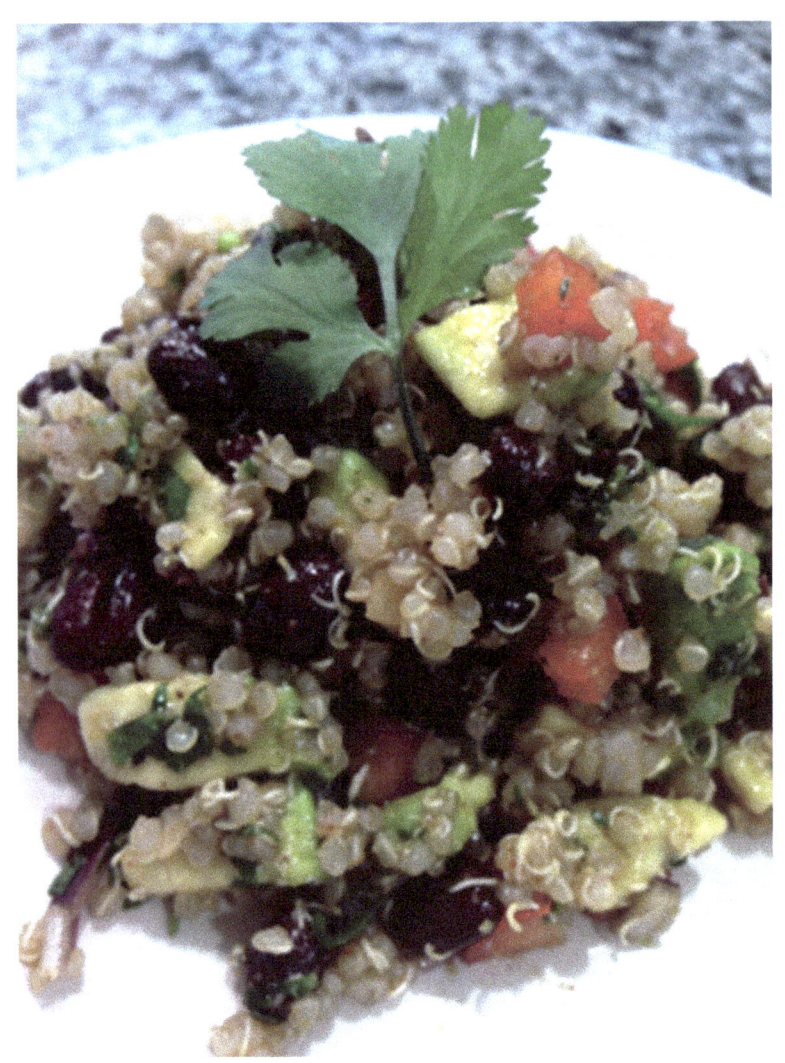

Quinoa and Black Bean Salad

Preparation time: 10 minutes
Cooking Time: 15 minutes + chilling time
Servings: 4
Ingredients:

- 2 cups water
- 1 cup quinoa, rinsed
- 16 ounces canned black beans, drained
- 2 Roma tomatoes, sliced
- 1 red onion, thinly sliced
- 1 cucumber, seeded and chopped
- 2 cloves garlic, pressed or minced
- 2 Italian peppers, seeded and sliced
- 2 tablespoons fresh parsley, chopped
- 2 tablespoons fresh cilantro, chopped
- 1/4 cup olive oil
- 1 lemon, freshly squeezed
- 1 tablespoon apple cider vinegar
- 1/2 teaspoon dried dill weed
- 1/2 teaspoon dried oregano
- Sea salt and ground black pepper, to taste

Directions:

1. Place the water and quinoa in a saucepan and bring it to a rolling boil. Immediately turn the heat to a simmer.
2. Let it simmer for about 13 minutes until the quinoa has absorbed all of the water; fluff the quinoa with a fork and let it cool completely. Then, transfer the quinoa to a salad bowl.
3. Add the remaining Ingredients to the salad bowl and toss to combine well. Bon appétit!

Nutrition: Calories: 433; Fat: 17.3g; Carbs: 57g; Protein: 15.1g

Rich Bulgur Salad with Herbs

Preparation time: 10 minutes
Cooking Time: 20 minutes + chilling time
Servings: 4
Ingredients:

- 2 cups water
- 1 cup bulgur
- 12 ounces canned chickpeas, drained
- 1 Persian cucumber, thinly sliced
- 2 bell peppers, seeded and thinly sliced
- 1 jalapeno pepper, seeded and thinly sliced
- 2 Roma tomatoes, sliced
- 1 onion, thinly sliced
- 2 tablespoons fresh basil, chopped
- 2 tablespoons fresh parsley, chopped
- 2 tablespoons fresh mint, chopped
- 2 tablespoons fresh chives, chopped
- 4 tablespoons olive oil
- 1 tablespoon balsamic vinegar
- 1 tablespoon lemon juice
- 1 teaspoon fresh garlic, pressed
- Sea salt and freshly ground black pepper, to taste
- 2 tablespoons nutritional yeast
- 1/2 cup Kalamata olives, sliced

Directions:

1. In a saucepan, bring the water and bulgur to a boil. Immediately turn the heat to a simmer and let it cook for about 20 minutes or until the bulgur is tender and water is almost absorbed. Fluff with a fork and spread on a large tray to let cool.

2. Place the bulgur in a salad bowl followed by the chickpeas, cucumber, peppers, tomatoes, onion, basil, parsley, mint and chives.
3. In a small mixing dish, whisk the olive oil, balsamic vinegar, lemon juice, garlic, salt and black pepper. Dress the salad and toss to combine.
4. Sprinkle nutritional yeast over the top, garnish with olives and serve at room temperature. Bon appétit!

Nutrition: Calories: 408; Fat: 18.3g; Carbs: 51.8g; Protein: 13.1g

Classic Roasted Pepper Salad

Preparation time: 10 minutes
Cooking Time: 15 minutes + chilling time
Servings: 3
Ingredients:

- 6 bell peppers
- 3 tablespoons extra-virgin olive oil
- 3 teaspoons red wine vinegar
- 3 garlic cloves, finely chopped
- 2 tablespoons fresh parsley, chopped
- Sea salt and freshly cracked black pepper, to taste
- 1/2 teaspoon red pepper flakes
- 6 tablespoons pine nuts, roughly chopped

Directions:

1. Broil the peppers on a parchment-lined baking sheet for about 10 minutes, rotating the pan halfway through the cooking time, until they are charred on all sides.
2. Then, cover the peppers with a plastic wrap to steam. Discard the skin, seeds and cores.
3. Slice the peppers into strips and toss them with the remaining ingredients. Place in your refrigerator until ready to serve. Bon appétit!

Nutrition: Calories: 178; Fat: 14.4g; Carbs: 11.8g; Protein: 2.4g

Hearty Winter Quinoa Soup

Preparation time: 10 minutes
Cooking Time: 25 minutes
Servings: 4
Ingredients:

- 2 tablespoons olive oil
- 1 onion, chopped
- 2 carrots, peeled and chopped
- 1 parsnip, chopped
- 1 celery stalk, chopped
- 1 cup yellow squash, chopped
- 4 garlic cloves, pressed or minced
- 4 cups roasted vegetable broth
- 2 medium tomatoes, crushed
- 1 cup quinoa
- Sea salt and ground black pepper, to taste
- 1 bay laurel
- 2 cup Swiss chard, tough ribs removed and torn into pieces
- 2 tablespoons Italian parsley, chopped

Directions:

1. In a heavy-bottomed pot, heat the olive over medium-high heat. Now, sauté the onion, carrot, parsnip, celery and yellow squash for about 3 minutes or until the vegetables are just tender.
2. Add in the garlic and continue to sauté for 1 minute or until aromatic.
3. Then, stir in the vegetable broth, tomatoes, quinoa, salt, pepper and bay laurel; bring to a boil. Immediately reduce the heat to a simmer and let it cook for 13 minutes.

4. Fold in the Swiss chard; continue to simmer until the chard wilts.
5. Ladle into individual bowls and serve garnished with the fresh parsley. Bon appétit!

Nutrition: Calories: 328; Fat: 11.1g; Carbs: 44.1g; Protein: 13.3g

Green Lentil Salad

Preparation time: 10 minutes
Cooking Time: 20 minutes + chilling time
Servings: 5
Ingredients:

- 1 ½ cups green lentils, rinsed
- 2 cups arugula
- 2 cups Romaine lettuce, torn into pieces
- 1 cup baby spinach
- 1/4 cup fresh basil, chopped
- 1/2 cup shallots, chopped
- 2 garlic cloves, finely chopped
- 1/4 cup oil-packed sun-dried tomatoes, rinsed and chopped
- 5 tablespoons extra-virgin olive oil
- 3 tablespoons fresh lemon juice
- Sea salt and ground black pepper, to taste

Directions:

1. In a large-sized saucepan, bring 4 ½ cups of the water and red lentils to a boil.
2. Immediately turn the heat to a simmer and continue to cook your lentils for a further 15 to 17 minutes or until they've softened but not mushy. Drain and let it cool completely.
3. Transfer the lentils to a salad bowl; toss the lentils with the remaining Ingredients until well combined.
4. Serve chilled or at room temperature. Bon appétit!

Nutrition: Calories: 349; Fat: 15.1g; Carbs: 40.9g; Protein: 15.4g

Acorn Squash, Chickpea and Couscous Soup

Preparation time: 10 minutes
Cooking Time: 20 minutes
Servings: 4
Ingredients:

- 2 tablespoons olive oil
- 1 shallot, chopped
- 1 carrot, trimmed and chopped
- 2 cups acorn squash, chopped
- 1 stalk celery, chopped
- 1 teaspoon garlic, finely chopped
- 1 teaspoon dried rosemary, chopped
- 1 teaspoon dried thyme, chopped
- 2 cups cream of onion soup
- 2 cups water
- 1 cup dry couscous
- Sea salt and ground black pepper, to taste
- 1/2 teaspoon red pepper flakes
- 6 ounces canned chickpeas, drained
- 2 tablespoons fresh lemon juice

Directions:

1. In a heavy-bottomed pot, heat the olive over medium-high heat. Now, sauté the shallot, carrot, acorn squash and celery for about 3 minutes or until the vegetables are just tender.
2. Add in the garlic, rosemary and thyme and continue to sauté for 1 minute or until aromatic.
3. Then, stir in the soup, water, couscous, salt, black pepper and red pepper flakes; bring to a

boil. Immediately reduce the heat to a simmer and let it cook for 12 minutes.
4. Fold in the canned chickpeas; continue to simmer until heated through or about 5 minutes more.
5. Ladle into individual bowls and drizzle with the lemon juice over the top. Bon appétit!

Nutrition: Calories: 378; Fat: 11g; Carbs: 60.1g; Protein: 10.9g

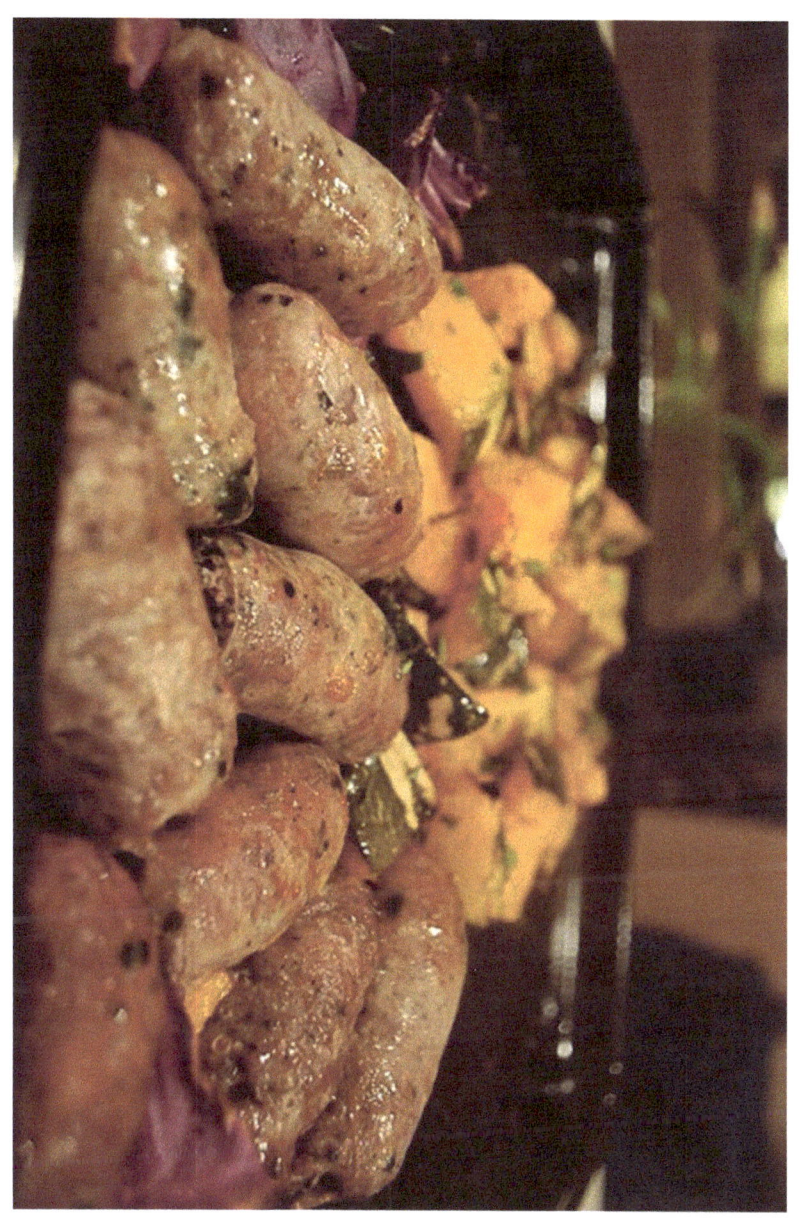

Cabbage Soup with Garlic Crostini

Preparation time: 10 minutes
Cooking Time: 1 hour
Servings: 4
Ingredients:

Soup:
- 2 tablespoons olive oil
- 1 medium leek, chopped
- 1 cup turnip, chopped
- 1 parsnip, chopped
- 1 carrot, chopped
- 2 cups cabbage, shredded
- 2 garlic cloves, finely chopped
- 4 cups vegetable broth
- 2 bay leaves
- Sea salt and ground black pepper, to taste
- 1/4 teaspoon cumin seeds
- 1/2 teaspoon mustard seeds
- 1 teaspoon dried basil
- 2 tomatoes, pureed

Crostini:
- 8 slices of baguette
- 2 heads garlic
- 4 tablespoons extra-virgin olive oil

Directions:

1. In a soup pot, heat 2 tablespoons of the olive over medium-high heat. Now, sauté the leek, turnip, parsnip and carrot for about 4 minutes or until the vegetables are crisp-tender.

2. Add in the garlic and cabbage and continue to sauté for 1 minute or until aromatic.
3. Then, stir in the vegetable broth, bay leaves, salt, black pepper, cumin seeds, mustard seeds, dried basil and pureed tomatoes; bring to a boil. Immediately reduce the heat to a simmer and let it cook for about 20 minutes.
4. Meanwhile, preheat your oven to 375 degrees F. Now, roast the garlic and baguette slices for about 15 minutes. Remove the crostini from the oven.
5. Continue baking the garlic for 45 minutes more or until very tender. Allow the garlic to cool.
6. Now, cut each head of the garlic using a sharp serrated knife in order to separate all the cloves.
7. Squeeze the roasted garlic cloves out of their skins. Mash the garlic pulp with 4 tablespoons of the extra-virgin olive oil.
8. Spread the roasted garlic mixture evenly on the tops of the crostini. Serve with the warm soup. Bon appétit!

Nutrition: Calories: 408; Fat: 23.1g; Carbs: 37.6g; Protein: 11.8g

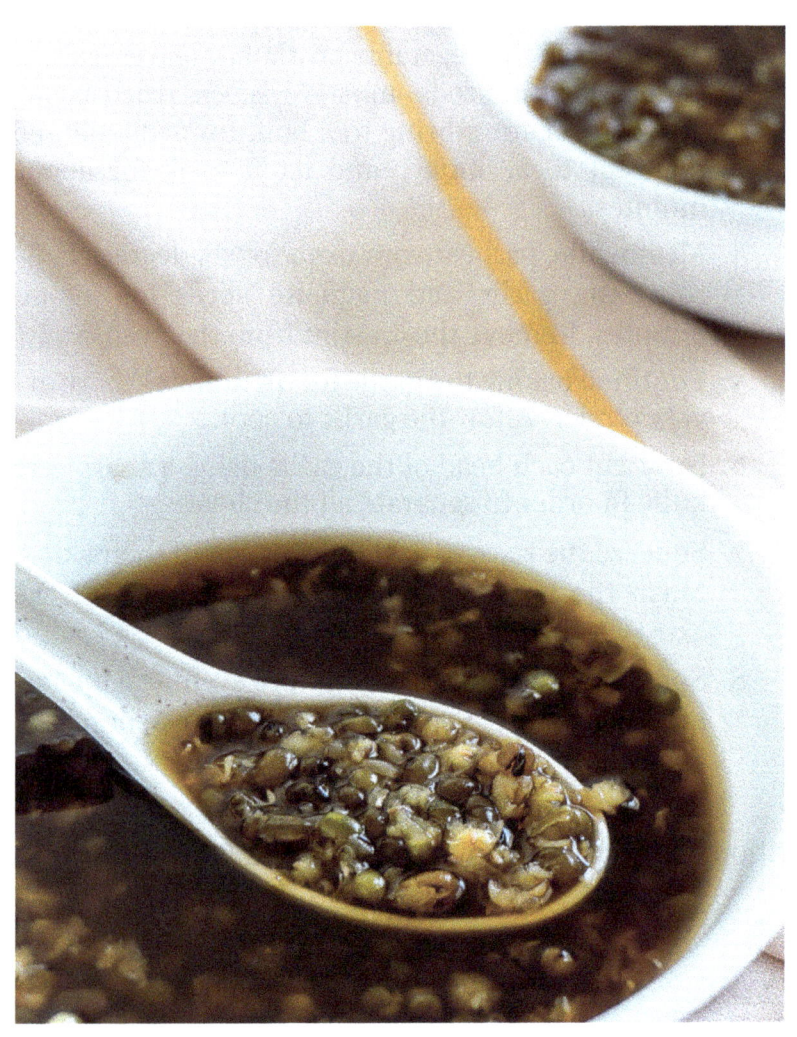

Cream of Green Bean Soup

Preparation time: 10 minutes
Cooking Time: 35 minutes
Servings: 4
Ingredients:

- 1 tablespoon sesame oil
- 1 onion, chopped
- 1 green pepper, seeded and chopped
- 2 russet potatoes, peeled and diced
- 2 garlic cloves, chopped
- 4 cups vegetable broth
- 1-pound green beans, trimmed
- Sea salt and ground black pepper, to season
- 1 cup full-fat coconut milk

Directions:

1. In a heavy-bottomed pot, heat the sesame over medium-high heat. Now, sauté the onion, peppers and potatoes for about 5 minutes, stirring periodically.
2. Add in the garlic and continue sautéing for 1 minute or until fragrant.
3. Then, stir in the vegetable broth, green beans, salt and black pepper; bring to a boil. Immediately reduce the heat to a simmer and let it cook for 20 minutes.
4. Puree the green bean mixture using an immersion blender until creamy and uniform.
5. Return the pureed mixture to the pot. Fold in the coconut milk and continue to simmer until heated through or about 5 minutes longer.
6. Ladle into individual bowls and serve hot. Bon appétit!

Nutrition: Calories: 410; Fat: 19.6g; Carbs: 50.6g; Protein: 13.3g

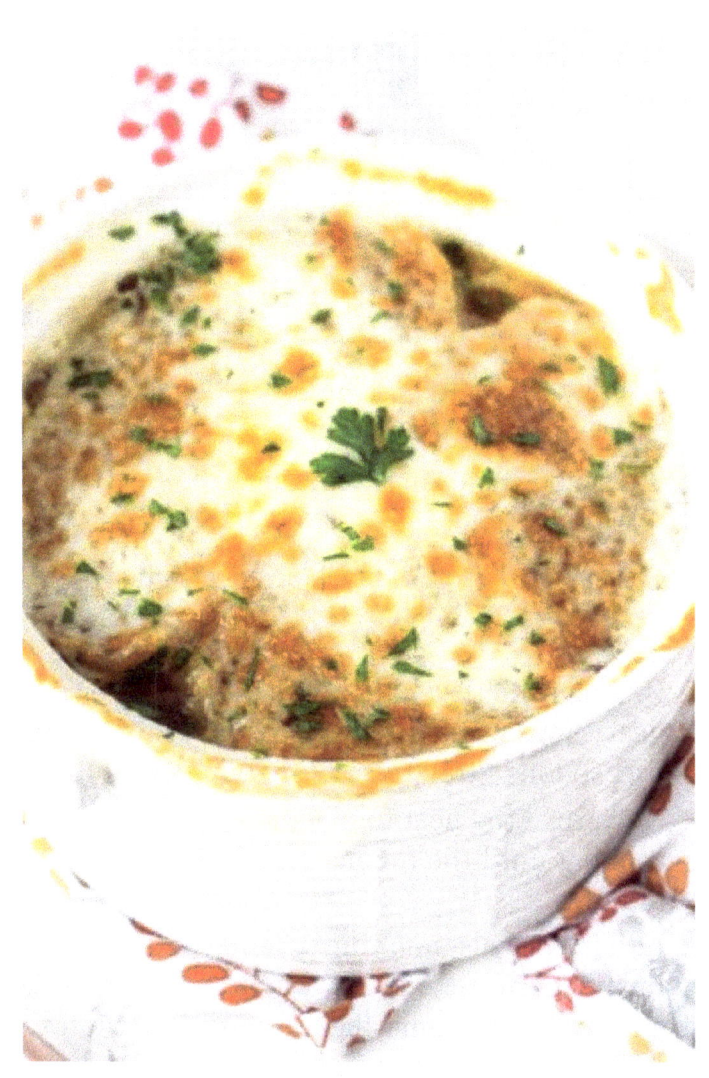

Traditional French Onion Soup

Preparation time: 10 minutes
Cooking Time: 1 hour 30 minutes
Servings: 4
Ingredients:

- 2 tablespoons olive oil
- 2 large yellow onions, thinly sliced
- 2 thyme sprigs, chopped
- 2 rosemary sprigs, chopped
- 2 teaspoons balsamic vinegar
- 4 cups vegetable stock
- Sea salt and ground black pepper, to taste

Directions:

1. In a or Dutch oven, heat the olive oil over a moderate heat. Now, cook the onions with thyme, rosemary and 1 teaspoon of the sea salt for about 2 minutes.
2. Now, turn the heat to medium-low and continue cooking until the onions caramelize or about 50 minutes.
3. Add in the balsamic vinegar and continue to cook for a further 15 more. Add in the stock, salt and black pepper and continue simmering for 20 to 25 minutes.
4. Serve with toasted bread and enjoy!

Nutrition: Calories: 129; Fat: 8.6g; Carbs: 7.4g; Protein: 6.3g

Roasted Carrot Soup

Preparation time: 10 minutes
Cooking Time: 50 minutes
Servings: 4
Ingredients:

- 1 ½ pounds carrots
- 4 tablespoons olive oil
- 1 yellow onion, chopped
- 2 cloves garlic, minced
- 1/3 teaspoon ground cumin
- Sea salt and white pepper, to taste
- 1/2 teaspoon turmeric powder
- 4 cups vegetable stock
- 2 teaspoons lemon juice
- 2 tablespoons fresh cilantro, roughly chopped

Directions:

1. Start by preheating your oven to 400 degrees F. Place the carrots on a large parchment-lined baking sheet; toss the carrots with 2 tablespoons of the olive oil.
2. Roast the carrots for about 35 minutes or until they've softened.
3. In a heavy-bottomed pot, heat the remaining 2 tablespoons of the olive oil. Now, sauté the onion and garlic for about 3 minutes or until aromatic.
4. Add in the cumin, salt, pepper, turmeric, vegetable stock and roasted carrots. Continue to simmer for 12 minutes more.
5. Puree your soup with an immersion blender. Drizzle lemon juice over your soup and serve garnished with fresh cilantro leaves. Bon appétit!

Nutrition: Calories: 264; Fat: 18.6g; Carbs: 20.1g; Protein: 7.4g

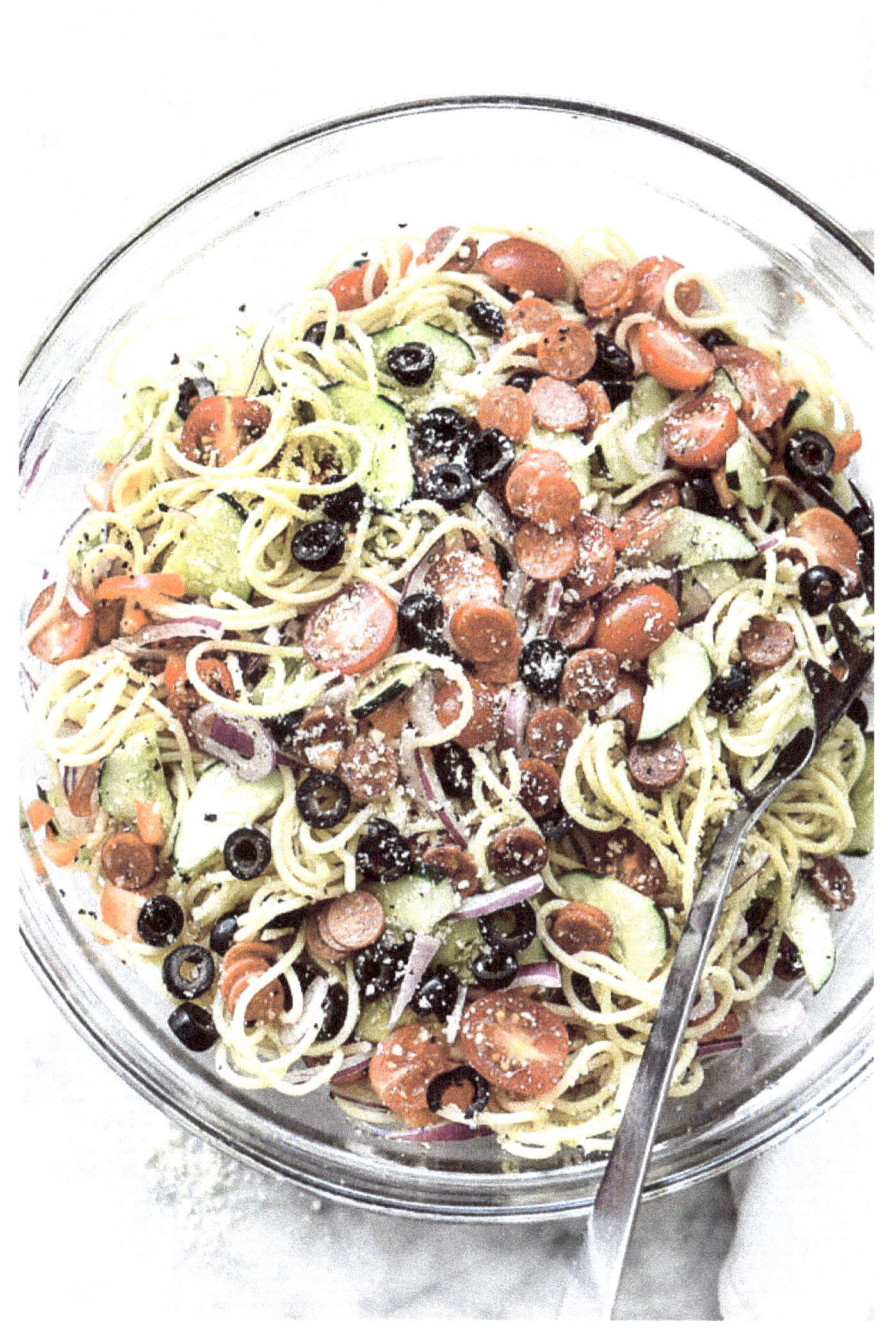

Italian Penne Pasta Salad

Preparation time: 10 minutes
Cooking Time: 15 minutes + chilling time
Servings: 3
Ingredients:

- 9 ounces penne pasta
- 9 ounces canned Cannellini bean, drained
- 1 small onion, thinly sliced
- 1/3 cup Niçoise olives, pitted and sliced
- 2 Italian peppers, sliced
- 1 cup cherry tomatoes, halved
- 3 cups arugula
- Dressing:
- 3 tablespoons extra-virgin olive oil
- 1 teaspoon lemon zest
- 1 teaspoon garlic, minced
- 3 tablespoons balsamic vinegar
- 1 teaspoon Italian herb mix
- Sea salt and ground black pepper, to taste

Directions:

1. Cook the penne pasta according to the package Directions. Drain and rinse the pasta. Let it cool completely and then, transfer it to a salad bowl.
2. Then, add the beans, onion, olives, peppers, tomatoes and arugula to the salad bowl.
3. Mix all the dressing Ingredients until everything is well incorporated. Dress your salad and serve well-chilled. Bon appétit!

Nutrition: Calories: 614; Fat: 18.1g; Carbs: 101g; Protein: 15.4g

Arugula with Fruits and Nuts

Preparation Time: 10 Minutes

Cooking Time: 0 Minutes

Servings: 1

Ingredients:

- ½ cup arugula
- ½ peach
- ½ red onion
- ¼ cup blueberries
- 5 walnuts, chopped
- 1 tbsp. extra-virgin olive oil
- 2 tbsp. red wine vinegar
- 1 spring of fresh basil

Directions:

1. Halve the peach and remove the seed. Heat a grill pan and grill it briefly on both sides. Cut the red onion into thin half-rings. Roughly chop the pecans.
2. Heat a pan and roast the pecans in it until they are fragrant.
3. Place the arugula on a plate and spread peaches, red onions, blueberries, and roasted pecans over it.
4. Put all the ingredients for the dressing in a food processor and mix to an even dressing. Drizzle the dressing over the salad.

Nutrition:

Calories: 160

Fat: 7g

Carbohydrate: 25g

Protein: 3g

Broccoli Salad

Preparation Time: 25 Minutes

Cooking Time: 0 Minutes

Servings: 2

Ingredients:

- 1 head of broccoli
- 1/2 red onion
- 2 carrots, grated
- ¼ cup red grapes
- 2 1/2 tbsp. Coconut yogurt
- 1 tbsp. Water
- 1 tsp. mustard
- 1 pinch salt

Directions:

1. Cut the broccoli into florets and cook for 8 minutes. Cut the red onion into thin half-rings. Halve the grapes. Mix coconut yogurt, water, and mustard with a pinch of salt to make the dressing.
2. Drain the broccoli and rinse with ice-cold water to stop the cooking process.
3. Mix the broccoli with the carrot, onion, and red grapes in a bowl. Serve the dressing separately on the side.

Nutrition:

Calories: 230

Fat: 18g

Carbohydrate: 35g

Protein: 10g

Brunoise Salad

Preparation Time: 10 Minutes

Cooking Time: 0 Minutes

Servings: 2

Ingredients:

- 1 tomato
- 1 zucchini
- ½ red bell pepper
- ½ yellow bell pepper
- ½ red onion
- 3 springs fresh parsley
- ½ lemon
- 2 tbsp. olive oil

Directions:

1. Finely dice tomatoes, zucchini, peppers, and red onions to get a brunoise. Mix all the cubes in a bowl. Chop parsley and mix in the salad. Squeeze the lemon over the salad and add the olive oil.
2. Season with salt and pepper.

Nutrition:

Calories: 84

Carbohydrate: 3g

Fat: 4g

Protein: 0g

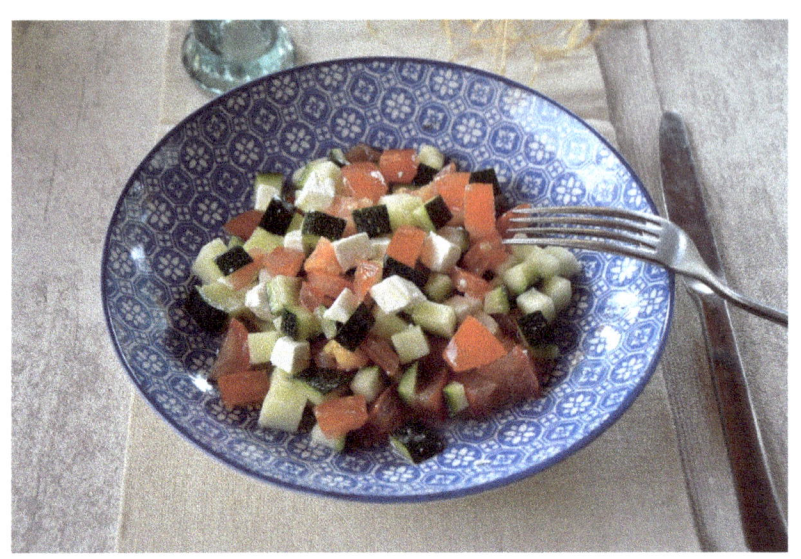

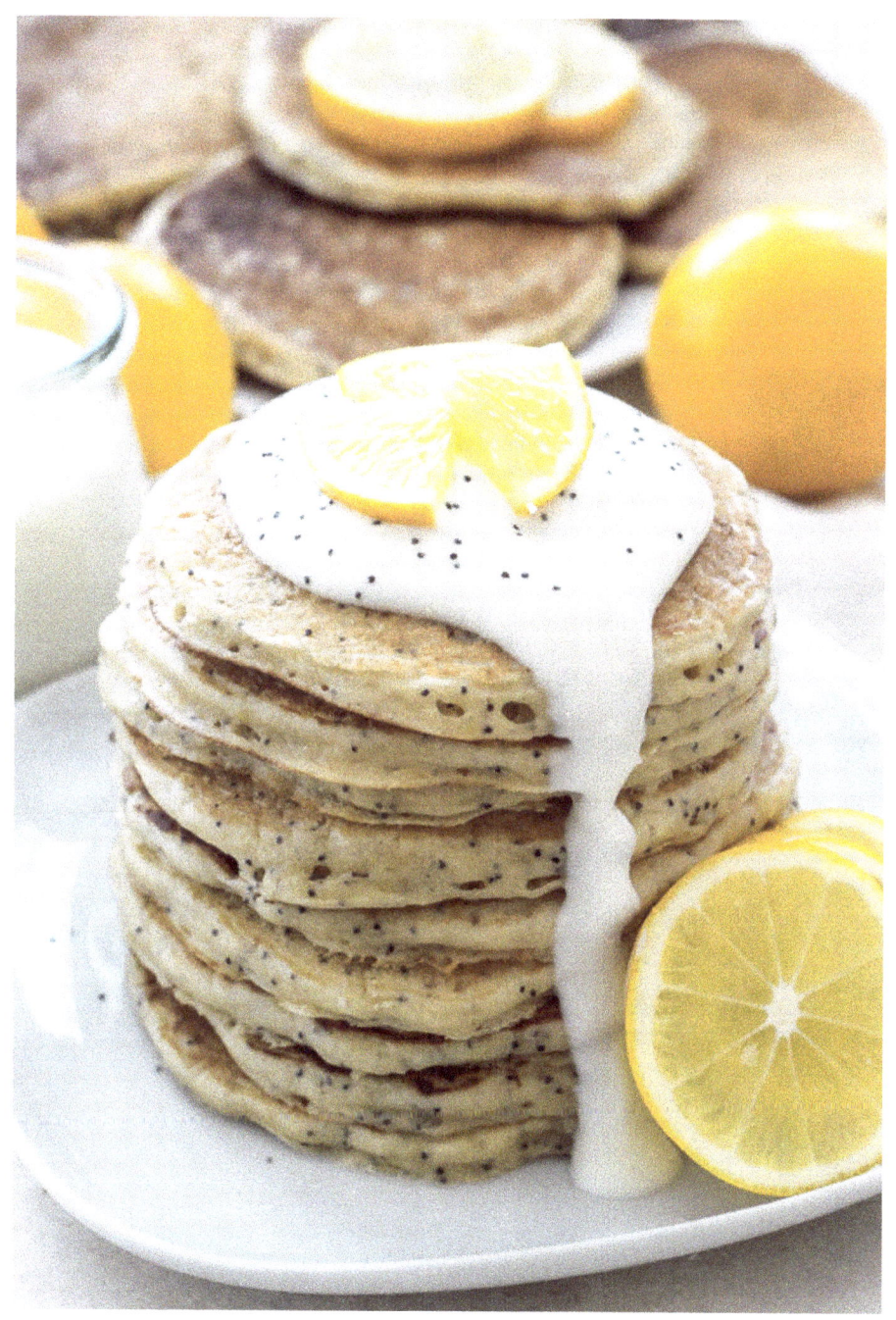

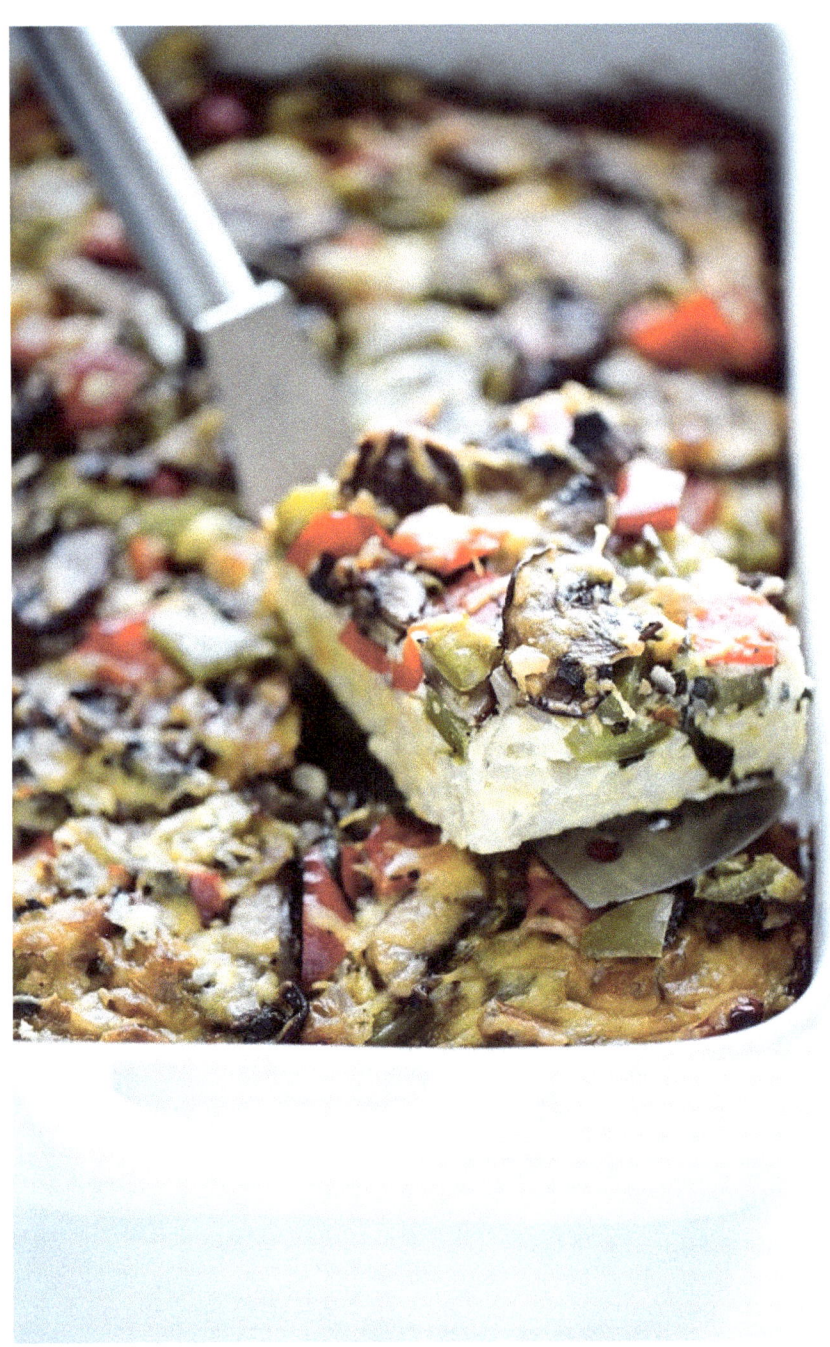

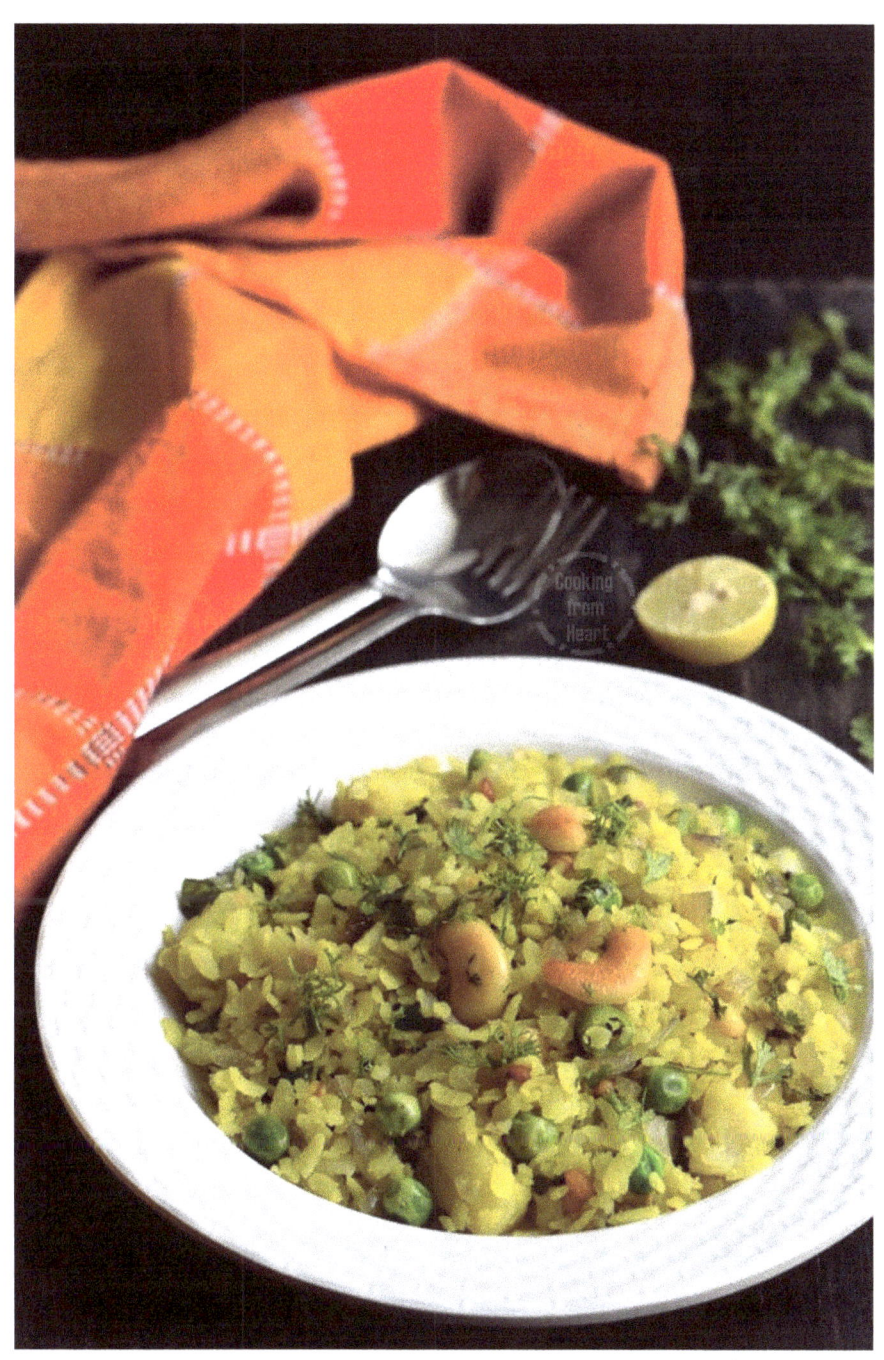

Breakfast Sandwich

Preparation Time: 5 Minutes

Cooking Time: 5 Minutes

Servings: 2

Ingredients:

- 3.5 oz. pumpkin flesh, peeled
- 4 slices whole grain bread
- 1 small avocado, pitted and peeled
- 1 carrot, finely grated
- 1 lettuce leaf, torn into four pieces

Directions:
Put pumpkin in a tray, introduce in the oven at 350 degrees and bake for 10 minutes.
1. Take pumpkin out of the oven, leave aside for 2-3 minutes, transfer to a bowl and mash it a bit
2. Put avocado in another bowl and also mash it with a fork.
3. Spread avocado on two bread slices, add grated carrot, mashed pumpkin and two lettuce pieces on each and top them with the rest of the bread slices.
4. Enjoy!

Nutrition:

Calories: 340

Fat: 7g

Carbs: 13g

Protein: 4g

Fiber: 8g

Sugar: 1g

Turkey Breakfast Sandwich

Preparation Time: 5 Minutes

Cooking Time: 5 Minutes

Servings: 1

Ingredients:

- 2 oz. turkey meat, roasted and thinly sliced
- 2 tbsp. pecans, toasted and chopped
- 2 oz. Brie cheese, sliced
- 2 slices sourdough bread
- 2 tbsp. cranberry chutney
- ¼ cup arugula

Directions:

1. In a bowl, mix pecans with chutney and stir well.
2. Spread this on bread slice, add turkey slices, brie cheese and arugula and top with the other bread slice.
3. Serve right away.
4. Enjoy!

Nutrition:

Calories: 100

Fat: 11g

Carbs: 52g

Protein: 32g

Fiber: 4g

Sugar: 0g

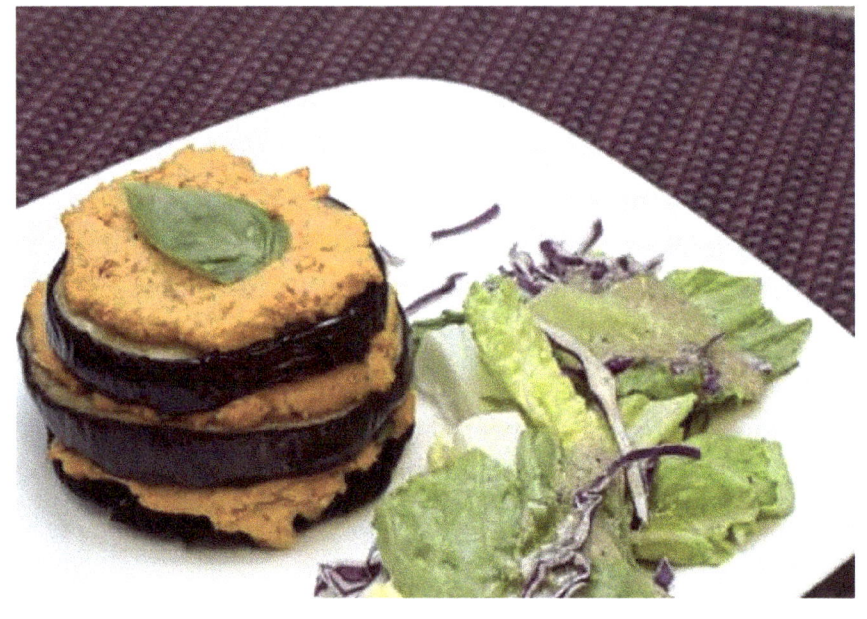

Eggplant Breakfast Spread

Preparation Time: 5 Minutes
Cooking Time: 15 Minutes
Servings: 2
Ingredients:

- 4 tbsp. olive oil
  2 lb. eggplants, peeled and roughly chopped
- 4 garlic cloves, minced
- A pinch of salt and black pepper
- 1 cup water
- ¼ cup lemon juice
- 1 tbsp. sesame seeds paste
- ¼ cup black olives, pitted
- A few sprigs thyme, chopped
- A drizzle of olive oil

Directions:

1. Set your instant pot on sauté mode, add oil, heat it up, add eggplant pieces, stir and sauté for 5 minutes
2. Add garlic, salt, pepper and the water, stir gently, cover and cook on High for 5 minutes.
3. Discard excess water, add sesame seeds paste, lemon juice and olives and blend using an immersion blender.
4. Transfer to a bowl, sprinkle chopped thyme, drizzle some oil and serve for a fancy breakfast.

Nutrition:

Calories: 163

Fat: 2g

Carbs: 5g

Protein: 7g

Fiber: 1g

Sugar: 0g

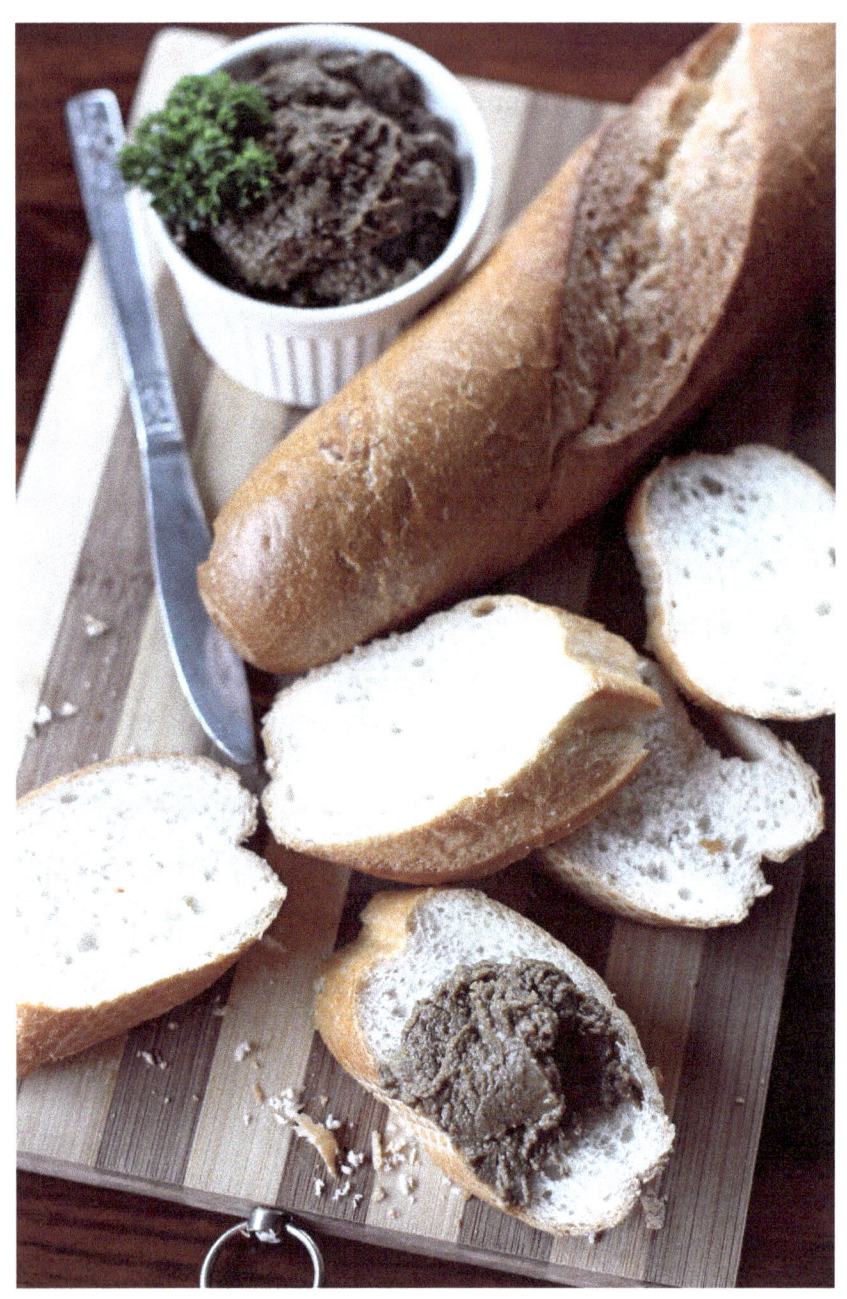

Chicken Liver Breakfast Spread

Preparation Time: 5 Minutes

Cooking Time: 15 Minutes

Servings: 2

Ingredients:

- 1 tsp. olive oil
- ¾ lb. chicken livers
- 1 yellow onion, chopped
- ¼ cup water
- 1 bay leaf
- 2 anchovies
- 1 tbsp. capers
- 1 tbsp. ghee
- A pinch of salt and black pepper

Directions:

1. Put the olive oil in your instant pot, add onion, salt, pepper, chicken livers, water and the bay leaf, stir, cover and cook on high for 10 minutes.
2. Discard bay leaf, add anchovies, capers and the ghee and pulse everything using your immersion blender.
3. Add salt and pepper, blend again, divide into bowls and serve for breakfast.

Nutrition:

Calories: 152

Fat: 4g

Carbs: 3g

Protein: 7g
Fiber: 2g

Sugar: 0g

Mushroom Spread

Preparation Time: 5 Minutes

Cooking Time: 25 Minutes

Servings: 2

Ingredients:

- 1 oz. porcini mushrooms, dried
- 1 lb. button mushrooms, sliced
- 1 cup hot water
- 1 tbsp. ghee
- 1 tbsp. olive oil
- 1 shallot, chopped
- ¼ cup cold water
- A pinch of salt and pepper
- 1 bay leaf

Directions:

1. Put porcini mushrooms in a bowl, add 1 cup hot water and leave aside for now.
2. Set your instant pot on sauté mode, add ghee and oil and heat it up.
3. Add shallot, stir and sauté for 2 minutes
4. Add porcini mushrooms and their liquid, fresh mushrooms, cold, salt, pepper and bay leaf, stir, cover and cook on high for 12 minutes,
5. Discard bay leaf and some of the liquid and blend mushrooms mix using an immersion blender.
6. Transfer to small bowls and serve as a breakfast spread.

Nutrition:

Calories: 120

Fat: 1g

Carbs: 1g

Protein: 10g

Fiber: 3g

Sugar: 0g

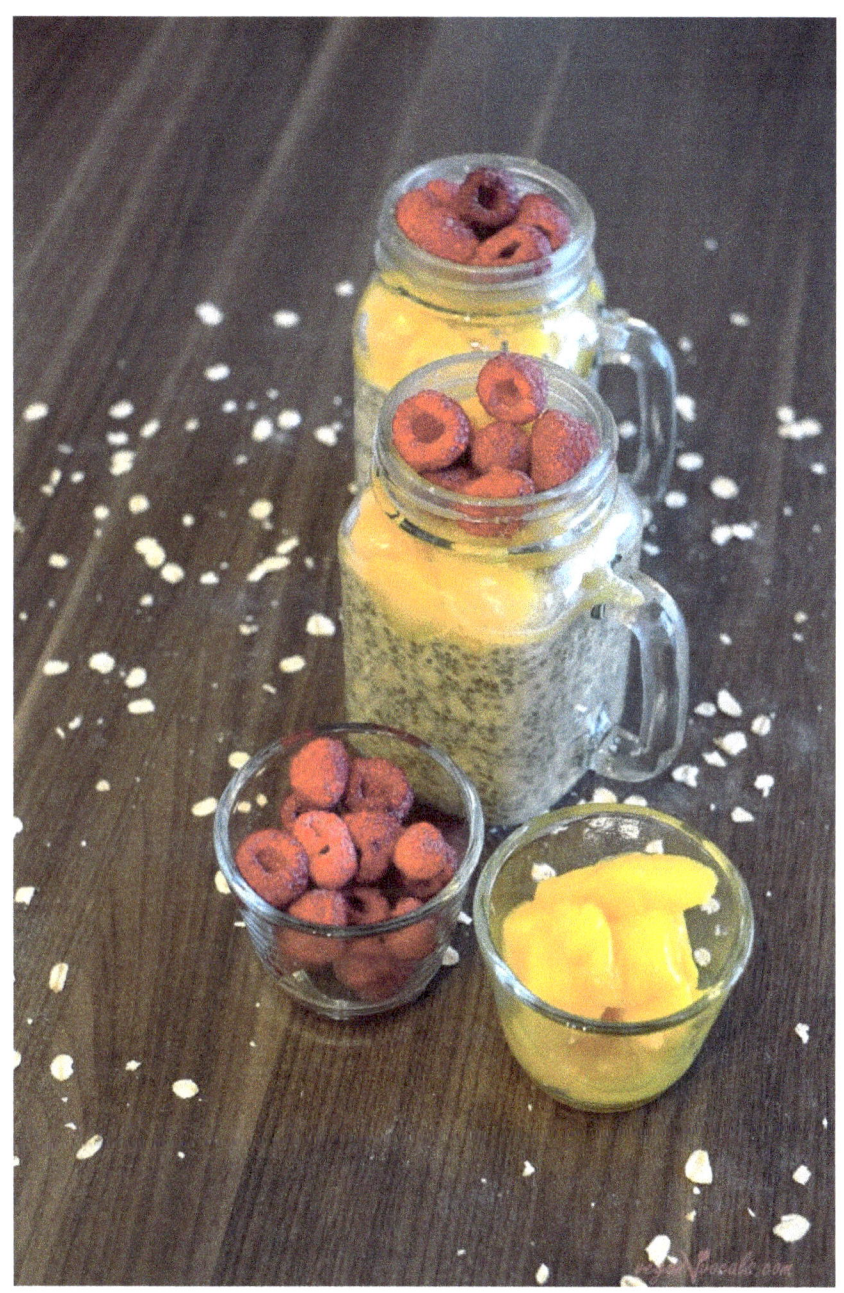

Breakfast Chia Pudding

Preparation Time: 5 Minutes

Cooking Time: 5 Minutes

Servings: 2

Ingredients:

- ½ cup chia seeds
- 2 cups almond milk
- ¼ cup almonds
- ¼ cup coconut, shredded
- 4 tsp. sugar

Directions:

1. Put chia seeds in your instant pot.
2. Add milk, almonds and coconut flakes, stir, cover and cook at high for 3 minutes
3. Release the pressure quick, divide the pudding between bowls, top each with a teaspoon of sugar and serve.

Nutrition:

Calories: 130

Fat: 1g

Carbs: 2g

Protein: 14g

Fiber: 5g

Sugar: 0g

Breakfast Sweet Potatoes

Preparation Time: 5 Minutes
Cooking Time: 15 Minutes
Servings: 2
Ingredients:

- 4 sweet potatoes
- 2 tsp. Italian seasoning
- 1 tbsp. bacon fat
- 1 cup chives, chopped for serving.
- Water
- Salt and pepper to taste

Directions:

1. Put potatoes in your instant pot, add water to cover them, cover the pot and cook at high for 10 minutes.
2. Release the pressure naturally, transfer potatoes to a working surface and leave them to cool down.
3. Peel potatoes, transfer them to a bowl and mash them a bit with a fork.
4. Set your instant pot on sauté mode, add bacon fat and heat up.
5. Add potatoes, seasoning, salt and pepper to the taste, stir, cover the pot and cook at high for 1 minute.
6. Release the pressure quickly, stir potatoes again, divide them between plates and serve with chives sprinkled on top.

Nutrition:

Calories: 90

Fat: 3g

Carbs: 6g

Protein: 7g

Fiber: 1g

Sugar: 0g

Eggs with Zucchini Noodles

Preparation Time: 10 Minutes
Cooking Time: 11 Minutes
Servings: 2
Ingredients:

- 2 tablespoons extra-virgin olive oil
- 3 zucchinis, cut with a spiralizer
- 4 eggs
  Salt and black pepper to the taste
- A pinch of red pepper flakes
- Cooking spray
- 1 tablespoon basil, chopped

Directions:

1. In a bowl, combine the zucchini noodles with salt, pepper, and the olive oil, and toss well.
2. Grease a baking sheet with cooking spray and divide the zucchini noodles into 4 nests on it.
3. Crack an egg on top of each nest, sprinkle salt, pepper, and the pepper flakes on top, and bake at 350 degrees F for 11 minutes.
4. Divide the mix between plates, sprinkle the basil on top, and serve.

Nutrition:

Calories: 296

Protein: 15 g

Fat: 24 g

Carbs: 11 g

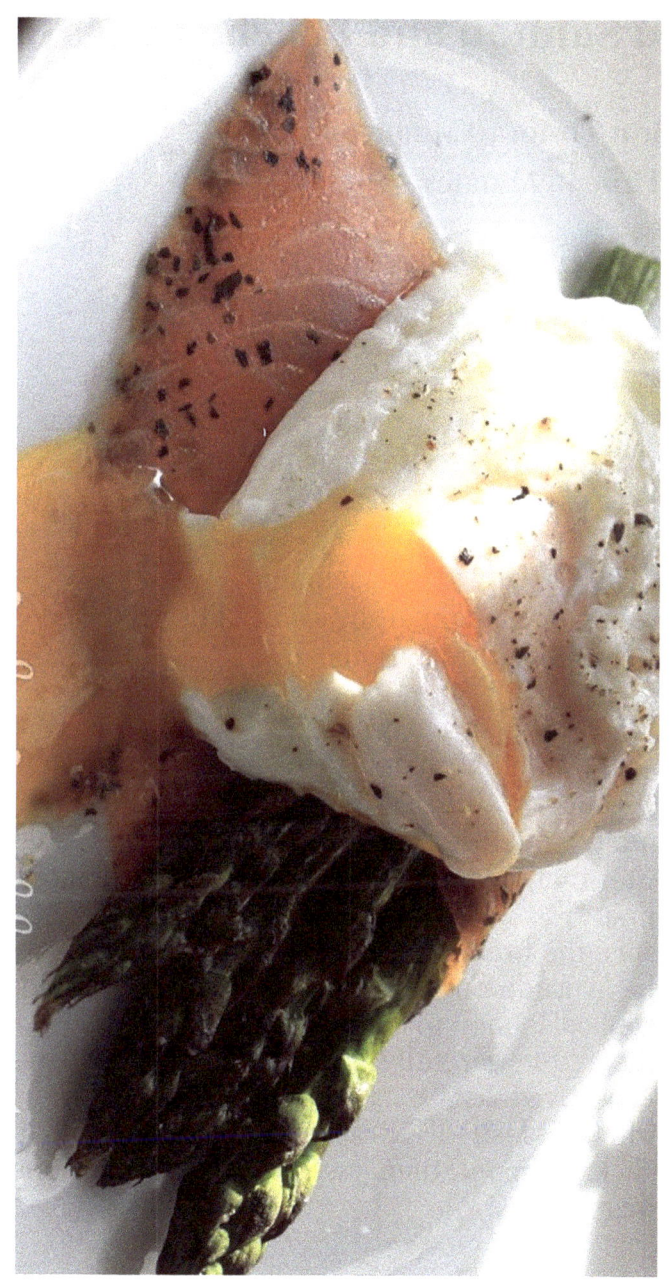

Smoked Salmon and Poached Eggs on Toast

Preparation Time: 10 Minutes

Cooking Time: 4 Minutes

Servings: 4

Ingredients:

- 2 oz avocado smashed
- 2 slices of bread toasted
- Pinch of kosher salt and cracked black pepper
- 1/4 tsp freshly squeezed lemon juice
- 2 eggs see notes, poached
- 3.5 oz smoked salmon
- 1 TBSP. thinly sliced scallions
- Splash of Kikkoman soy sauce optional
- Microgreens are optional

Directions:

1. Take a small bowl and then smash the avocado into it. Then, add the lemon juice and also a pinch of salt into the mixture. Then, mix it well and set aside.
2. After that, poach the eggs and toast the bread for some time.
3. Once the bread is toasted, you will have to spread the avocado on both slices and after that, add the smoked salmon to each slice.
4. Thereafter, carefully transfer the poached eggs to the respective toasts.
5. Add a splash of Kikkoman soy sauce and some cracked pepper; then, just garnish with scallions and microgreens.

Nutrition:

Calories: 459

Protein: 31 g

Fat: 22 g

Carbs: 33 g

Mediterranean Breakfast Salad

Preparation Time: 10 Minutes

Cooking Time: 20 Minutes

Servings: 4

Ingredients:

- 4 whole eggs
- 2 cups of cherry tomatoes or heirloom tomatoes cut in half or wedges
- 10 cups of arugula
- A 1/2 chopped seedless cucumber
- 1 large avocado
- 1 cup cooked or cooled quinoa
- 1/2 cup of chopped mixed herbs like dill and mint
- 1 cup of chopped Almonds
- 1 lemon
- extra virgin olive oil
- sea salt
- freshly ground black pepper

Directions:

1. In this recipe, the eggs are the first thing that needs to be cooked. Start with soft boiling the eggs. To do that, you need to get water in a pan and let it sit to boil. Once it starts boiling, reduces the heat to simmer and lower the eggs into the water and let them cook for about 6 minutes. After they are boiled, wash the eggs with cold water and set aside. Peel them when they are cool and ready to use.
2. Combine quinoa, arugula, cucumbers, and tomatoes in a bowl and add a little bit of olive oil over the top. Toss it with salt and pepper to equally season all of it.
3. Once all that is done, serve the salad on four plates and garnish it with sliced avocados and the halved eggs. After that, season it with some more pepper and salt.

4. To top it all off, then use almonds and sprinkle some herbs along with some lemon zest and olive oil.

Nutrition:

calories: 85

protein: 3.4 g

fat: 3.46 g

carbs: 6.71 g

Honey Almond Ricotta Spread with Peaches

Preparation Time: 5 Minutes

Cooking Time: 8 Minutes

Servings: 4

Ingredients:

- 1/2 cup Fisher Sliced Almonds
- 1 cup whole milk ricotta
- 1/4 teaspoon almond extract
- zest from an orange, optional
- 1 teaspoon honey
- hearty whole-grain toast
- English muffin or bagel
- extra Fisher sliced almonds
- sliced peaches
- extra honey for drizzling

Directions:

1. Cut peaches into a proper shape and then brush them with olive oil. After that, set it aside.
2. Take a bowl; combine the ingredients for the filling. Set aside.
3. Then just pre-heat grill to medium.
4. Place peaches cut side down onto the greased grill.
5. Close lid cover and then just grill until the peaches have softened, approximately 6-10 minutes, depending on the size of the peaches.
6. Then you will have to place peach halves onto a serving plate.
7. Put a spoon of about 1 tablespoon of ricotta mixture into the cavity (you are also allowed to use a small scooper).
8. Sprinkle it with slivered almonds, crushed amaretti cookies, and honey.
9. Decorate with the mint leaves.

Nutrition:

Calories: 187
Protein: 7 g
Fat: 9 g
Carbs: 18 g

Mediterranean Eggs Cups

Preparation Time: 10 Minutes

Cooking Time: 20 Minutes

Servings: 8

Ingredients:

- 1 cup spinach, finely diced
- 1/2 yellow onion, finely diced
- 1/2 cup sliced sun-dried tomatoes
- 4 large basil leaves, finely diced
- Pepper and salt to taste
- 1/3 cup feta cheese crumbles
- 8 large eggs
- 1/4 cup milk (any kind)

Directions:

1. You have to heat the oven to 375°F.
2. Then, roll the dough sheet into a 12x8-inch rectangle
3. Then, cut in half lengthwise
4. After that, you will have to cut each half crosswise into 4 pieces, forming 8 (4x3-inch) pieces dough. Then, press each into the bottom and up sides of the ungreased muffin cup.
5. Trim dough to keep the dough from touching, if essential. Set aside.
6. Then, you will have to combine the eggs, salt, pepper in the bowl and beat it with a whisk until well mixed. Set aside.
7. Melt the butter in 12-inch skillet over medium heat until sizzling; add bell peppers.
8. You will have to cook it, stirring occasionally, 2-3 minutes or until crisply tender.
9. After that, add spinach leaves; continue cooking until spinach is wilted. Then just add egg mixture and prosciutto.
10. Divide the mixture evenly among prepared muffin cups.

11. Finally, bake it for 14-17 minutes or until the crust is golden brown.

Nutrition:

Calories: 240

Protein: 9 g

Fat: 16 g

Carbs: 13 g

Low-Carb Baked Eggs with Avocado and Feta

Preparation Time: 10 Minutes

Cooking Time: 15 Minutes

Servings: 2

Ingredients:

- 1 avocado
- 4 eggs
- 2-3 tbsp. crumbled feta cheese
- Nonstick cooking spray
- Pepper and salt to taste

Directions:

1. First, you will have to preheat the oven to 400 degrees F.
2. After that, when the oven is on the proper temperature, you will have to put the gratin dishes right on the baking sheet.
3. Then, leave the dishes to heat in the oven for almost 10 minutes
4. After that process, you need to break the eggs into individual ramekins.
5. Then, let the avocado and eggs come to room temperature for at least 10 minutes
6. Then, peel the avocado properly and cut it each half into 6-8 slices
7. You will have to remove the dishes from the oven and spray them with the non-stick spray
8. Then, you will have to arrange all the sliced avocados in the dishes and tip two eggs into each dish
9. Sprinkle with feta, add pepper and salt to taste

Nutrition:

Calories: 280

Protein: 11 g

Fat: 23 g
Carbs: 10 g

Mediterranean Eggs White Breakfast Sandwich with Roasted Tomatoes

Preparation Time: 15 Minutes

Cooking Time: 10 Minutes

Servings: 2

Ingredients:

- Salt and pepper to taste
- ¼ cup egg whites
  1 teaspoon chopped fresh herbs like rosemary, basil,
- parsley,
- 1 whole-grain seeded ciabatta roll
- 1 teaspoon butter
- 1-2 slices Muenster cheese
- 1 tablespoon pesto
- About ½ cup roasted tomatoes
- 10 ounces grape tomatoes
- 1 tablespoon extra-virgin olive oil
- Black pepper and salt to taste

Directions:

1. First, you will have to melt the butter over medium heat in the small nonstick skillet.
2. Then, mix the egg whites with pepper and salt.
4. Then, sprinkle it with the fresh herbs
5. After that cook it for almost 3-4 minutes or until the eggs are done, then flip it carefully
6. Meanwhile, toast ciabatta bread in the toaster
7. After that, you will have to place the egg on the bottom half of the sandwich rolls, then top with cheese
8. Add roasted tomatoes and the top half of roll.
9. To make a roasted tomato, preheat the oven to 400 degrees.
10. Then, slice the tomatoes in half lengthwise.
    10. Place on the baking sheet and drizzle with olive oil.

11. Season it with pepper and salt and then roast in the oven for about 20 minutes. Skins will appear wrinkled when done.

Nutrition:

Calories: 458

Protein: 21 g

Fat: 24 g

Carbs: 51 g

Greek Yogurt Pancakes

Preparation Time: 10 Minutes

Cooking Time: 5 Minutes

Servings: 2

Ingredients:

- 1 cup all-purpose flour
- 1 cup whole-wheat flour
- 1/4 teaspoon salt
- 4 teaspoons baking powder
- 1 Tablespoon sugar
- 1 1/2 cups unsweetened almond milk
- 2 teaspoons vanilla extract
- 2 large eggs
- 1/2 cup plain 2% Greek yogurt
- Fruit, for serving
- Maple syrup, for serving

Directions:

1. First, you will have to pour the curds into the bowl and mix them well until creamy.
2. You will have to put egg whites then mix them well until combined.
3. Then take a distinct bowl, pour the wet mixture into the dry mixture. Stir to combine. The batter will be extremely thick.

4. Spoon the batter onto the sprayed pan heated to medium-high.
5. Then, you will have to flip the pancakes once when they begin to bubble a bit on the surface. Cook until golden brown on both sides.

Nutrition:

Calories: 166

Protein: 14 g

Fat: 5 g

Carbs: 52g

Mediterranean Feta and Quinoa Egg Muffins

Preparation Time: 15 Minutes

Cooking Time: 15 Minutes
Servings: 12

Ingredients:

- 2 cups baby spinach finely chopped
- 1 cup chopped or sliced cherry tomatoes
- 1/2 cup finely chopped onion
- 1 tablespoon chopped fresh oregano
- 1 cup crumbled feta cheese
- 1/2 cup chopped {pitted} kalamata olives
- 2 teaspoons high oleic sunflower oil
- 1 cup cooked quinoa
- 8 eggs
- 1/4 teaspoon salt

Directions:

1. Pre-heat oven to 350 degrees Fahrenheit
2. Make 12 silicone muffin holders on the baking sheet, or just grease a 12-cup muffin tin with oil and set aside.
3. Finely slice the vegetables
4. Heat the skillet to medium.
5. Add the vegetable oil and onions and sauté for 2 minutes.
6. Then, add tomatoes and sauté for another minute, then add spinach and sauté until wilted, about 1 minute.
7. Put the beaten egg into a bowl and then add lots of vegetables like feta cheese, quinoa, veggie mixture as well as salt, and then stir well until everything is properly combined.
8. Pour the ready mixture into greased muffin tins or silicone cups, dividing the mixture equally. Then, bake it in an oven for 30 minutes or so, or until the

eggs set nicely, and the muffins turn a light golden brown in color.

Nutrition:

Calories: 113

Protein: 6 g

Fat: 7 g

Carbs: 5 g

www.ingramcontent.com/pod-product-compliance
Lightning Source LLC
Chambersburg PA
CBHW071108030426
42336CB00013BA/2002